THE YEAR
I PRESSED PAUSE

My Journey with Breast Cancer

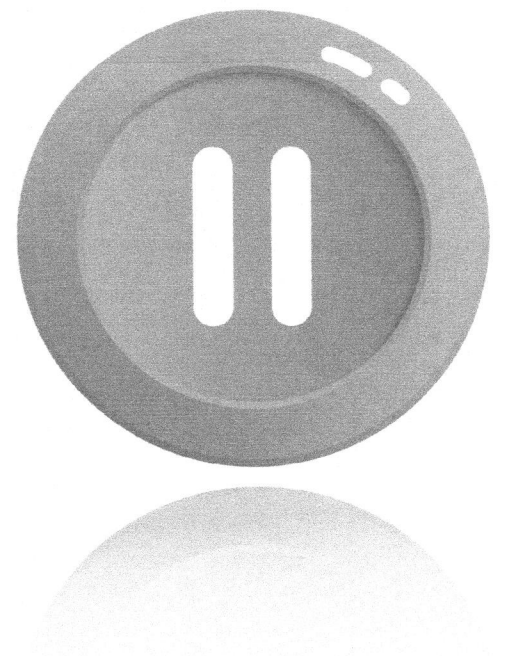

A MEMOIR BY

HEIDI SCHAFER-EDWARDS

The Year I Pressed Pause: My Journey with Breast Cancer
Heidi Schafer-Edwards

ISBN 978-1-66783-000-1

Contents

PROLOGUE

On July 5, 2017, I was diagnosed with Triple Negative Breast Cancer (TNBC). Nine days after diagnosis, I started posting updates on CaringBridge. Caringridge is a free on-line journal that allows users going through health crises to post updates for family and friends. In January of 2021 (in the midst of the COVID pandemic) I revisited these posts and decided to write an autobiographical narrative about my breast cancer journey. Essentially, the reader will find my initial post followed by my "reflection" on each post. While the initial posts are dated, the reflections are not. All of the reflections were written between January and September of 2021. The editing was done in October, November, and December, and the book was printed in early 2022. Some names have been changed to protect privacy.

FROM FEELING A LUMP TO RECEIVING A CANCER DIAGNOSIS

JOURNAL ENTRY BY HEIDI EDWARDS
JULY 14, 2017

At the beginning of June, I felt a small lump near my armpit on my left breast. I was concerned and I wanted to worry, but I decided to move that worry into action and called my primary care doctor, Dr. Kane. She was out of town that week, so I made an appointment for mid-June. After my visit with her, she recommended a mammogram and ultrasound. I was going to be on vacation with my sister-in-law and all the cousins (her three and my three) the following week, so I scheduled the imaging for June 26th. After the two exams, the radiologist who read the imaging felt like a biopsy was warranted. More waiting........ A biopsy was set up for Friday, June 30th. I arrived at the Breast Center on June 30th by 9:30 a.m., and by 11:00 a.m. I was back in the minivan with an ice pack in my bra and an Ace bandage wrapped around my chest. We headed up North for the long holiday weekend and kept ourselves distracted while we waited for "the call" on Wednesday. Wednesday morning the pathologist called Doug (he had spoken to her the previous Friday) and told us the pathology came back as invasive ductal carcinoma. She also shared that the cancer was an aggressive type and was growing quickly. As we left our cabin and drove home, the world felt like a much different place.

Reflection

Many of the breast cancer stories I have read start out like this:

I first felt the lump_____.

The above sentence is a prompt. As a person who has devoted a fair bit of her life to teaching writing, I recognize the value of a prompt. A prompt starts the writer off, gives the writer something to think about, a way to begin. In writing, sometimes beginning is the hardest part of the essay or paper or story. I think the beginning of a breast cancer journey is the hardest part as well. It is hard because there is so much UNCERTAINTY. The patient doesn't know the extent of the cancer. She doesn't know how the cancer will be treated. She doesn't know how the cancer will affect her partner, her family, her job, and on and on. She doesn't know if the cancer is survivable. I am using the word she while recognizing that men also face breast cancer diagnoses. I am inclusive of these men as I share my experiences even while using the pronoun she. I also recognize that not all breast cancer patients feel a lump. Some breast cancer is discovered on a mammogram. Advanced breast cancer might first be discovered when a patient has another complaint that ends up showing the breast cancer has spread beyond the lump.

I first felt "the lump" <u>in the shower.</u> (prompt response) I do not remember the exact date, but I know it was in early June of 2017. My nature is to be a bit of a hypochondriac, but for some reason I honestly wasn't overly worried when I felt the pea sized abnormality near the armpit of my left breast-at about ten o'clock. I called to make an appointment with my internist. She was on vacation, so I was not able to see her for a few weeks, in mid-June. In the time between feeling the lump and visiting the doctor, I would feel the spot periodically, just to see if it was still there. It never disappeared. When I finally saw Dr. Kane, she congratulated me on a twenty pound weight loss since my last visit. After a bit of chit-chat, she examined me sitting up and then laying down. She felt the lump, and ordered a mammogram and ultrasound. She also set up an appointment with a breast surgeon-"just in case". Her reasoning seemed solid.

"If there is something," she said, "I don't want you to have to wait a few weeks to see the surgeon. We can always cancel, but we can't get an appointment really quickly if there is something off. We will schedule the appointment with the breast surgeon 7-10 days after the mammogram and ultrasound. That way, if you end up needing a biopsy, the timing should work out so that you will see the surgeon right after you get the results from the biopsy. Women's health is usually pretty quick with setting up biopsies after the mammo and ultrasound if they think a biopsy is warranted."

I started to understand the process from feeling a lump to having a diagnosis. I hoped that the process for me would end with a mammogram and ultrasound and never go any further.

She never said the word cancer, even though that is what we were both most afraid of. I have a physician as a husband. I know that he is often afraid for his patients and sometimes fears the worst. He is occasionally in the business of ruling out the "worst". Dr. Kane's first priority was ruling out the worst.

I was taking an annual cousins' trip with my sister-in-law, Jody, to southwest Florida the next week, so the mammogram and diagnostic ultrasound got put off until the last week of June. Still, that deep worry that settles in the pit of your stomach during times of concern wasn't there. I enjoyed my vacation with Jody and our kiddos (six in total). When I look at the pictures from that trip now, I see a different version of myself. The 44-year-old woman in the photos wearing a polka dot Lands End swim cover up seems like someone I don't know. Her hair is longer and brown. She looks younger and more naive.

We came back from Florida on a Saturday, and on Monday, June 26th, I headed into Women's Health at a hospital in north central WI (where I live). The mammogram was scheduled first. A diagnostic mammogram is different from a preventative mammogram. The technician met with me before and marked (with a marker) the spot I had felt. After the mammogram, I had a breast ultrasound. Unfortunately, this was not my first ultrasound. Five years earlier, in 2012, I had a bout with thyroid cancer. I had a number of ultrasounds during treatment for that health situation. I also had a twin pregnancy and a twin birth, so I was no stranger to the goopy, clear liquid/solid, the robe that opens in the front, the dark room and the waiting afterwards while the technician "makes sure the doctor has enough pictures".

Following the completion of both exams, the radiologist actually came in and met with me. He told me they had enough images, but explained that more testing was needed and discussed performing a biopsy.

I left the discussion with the radiologist and met with an RN who was given the title of Nurse Navigator. Because we were nearing the July 4th holiday, timing was a bit tricky. Unfortunately, the earliest biopsy appointment was Friday, June 30th. Normally, patients find out the results the day after the biopsy, except on Fridays when results are given on Mondays. But..... because of Tuesday being July 4th, I would not have my results until July 5th. That meant I would wait a full five days from biopsy to results. The nurse gave me the option of scheduling a biopsy for the 5th of July, but once I knew that the question of whether or not I had cancer was on the table, I chose the option that would answer that question most quickly— even if only by a day. I left the Center with a pink brochure titled "About Your Breast Biopsy" (or something like that) and a lot of anxiety.

Friday came after an anxious week of waiting and worrying - the sick, ever present anxious feeling was with me now. The only thing that would make that feeling go away was the news that the lump was benign. My appointment was in the morning. Doug, my physician husband, did not come with me because moving scheduled patients during a busy clinic day is hard. It is hard for the patients and their family members who may have taken time off work to attend an appointment with their mom or dad, their son or daughter. It is hard for the schedulers who, in his absence, have to call every single affected patient and reschedule. It is hard for the staff members who are scheduled to work with Doug. When he is gone, what do they do? And so.... in the way that I had attended almost all medical appointments up to this point in our marriage, I went alone.

Getting a biopsy is icky on so many levels. The patient is in a vulnerable, nervous state with people he or she doesn't know in a situation he or she has no reference for. After I checked in, I sat in the waiting area with other women, most of whom were waiting for yearly mammograms. Most of them did not look worried. I felt like I knew something they did not.

I wanted to warn them, but warn them about what? I thumbed through magazines without really reading anything.

After about ten minutes of waiting, I changed into a white bathrobe and left my top and bra in a locked locker with the key on a fob on my wrist. Then it was on to another waiting area where, after ten minutes, I followed another technician to a different room for an ultrasound. Once I was in position, she cleaned my breast, added the warm gel and navigated until she found the spot. She left me on the table with the white bathrobe and went to find the interventional radiologist who would do the biopsy. In a biopsy, the technician and the radiologist use ultrasound technology to find the area in question. Then, the radiologist takes a hollow needle to obtain several samples of the suspicious tissue. The radiologist had already numbed the area, so each time he took a sample, all I could feel was a strange pulling and pressure. It was over quickly and the radiologist left. He left a little metal marker in the spot where the biopsy was for future reference which I came to understand is standard procedure.

The technician left me in the care of the Nurse Navigator. She placed firm pressure on the spot where the biopsy had occurred for about ten minutes. This surprised me and seemed like an exaggerated response to the procedure. I wanted to say, "It's OK, no worries, I am fine." But I didn't say anything. I chatted with her to let her know that I was OK. Eventually, she bandaged the spot and then wrapped my chest with an ACE bandage. The last step in this process was the insertion of small ice packs between a few of the layers of the ACE bandage. Once I was all bandaged up, she invited me to follow her to the locker room. She waited outside while I put on my shirt, and then we walked together to her office.

"So, do you have any plans for the Fourth?" she asked while handing me a folder with information I wasn't interested in learning about.

Besides waiting to see if I have breast cancer, I wanted to ask.

"Well, we have a cabin Up North, so our plan is to be there," I responded instead.

"So, as we discussed when we made the appointment, we won't have your results until next Wednesday because of the holiday. We should call you right after lunch. That is when we usually get the results from pathology. Until then, you should not do any heavy lifting as it can cause a hematoma which is a collection of blood around the area of the biopsy. Try to ice as much as possible. Finally, try not to worry. Most biopsies are benign." She gave me a little pamphlet with a title on front that said something like "After Your Biopsy". I wondered if it was written by the same person who had written "Before Your Biopsy".

I walked through the lobby where more women were waiting to be called back, change into white robes, and follow a technician down a hall to a darkened room for their mammograms. It was bright when I opened the door and I blinked. Outside, it was just a normal Friday afternoon and the world was still spinning. Everything seemed surreal to me. It didn't seem like the world should be normal, but it was. I walked to my minivan and sat in the driver's seat for a while before I called Doug who picked up after just a few rings. He asked me lots of questions, but the recurrent theme was the same,

"Does the radiologist think that it is cancer?"

"He doesn't know, Doug, he didn't give me any indication one way or another. That is why they do the biopsy."

Doug knew that too. He had already talked to his BFF's from med school, one who was a pathologist and two who were themselves radiologists. One of these two even does a lot of breast imaging as part of his practice. He had shared the initial images with this friend who told him the same thing.

"It's suspicious, Doug, but you can't know without the biopsy."

And so we waited. The Friday after the biopsy we had a grad party for one of our best friends. Doug had to work, but the girls and I hopped back in the minivan and drove about thirty minutes to attend the party which was at the family's lake house. Everyone at the party was festive and happy, celebrating the graduate, but also gearing up for the 4th. Where we live, in north-central WI, the fourth of July is a big deal and lots and lots of people have places "Up North". Heading "Up North" means hopping on 51N for lots of folks and heading to places like Minocqua and Boulder Junction, Eagle River and 3 Lakes, St. Germain and Presque Isle. It means boating, eating, campfires, friends, 4th of July parades, and fireworks. It means an escape from everyday life—a time to let loose and relax.

Oftentimes, in the past, we have hosted friends or family for the holiday weekend, and I was thankful that was not the case this year. It would have been hard to keep all the worries and fear hidden behind a facade. It was just us, and I was grateful. The girls knew about the biopsy, but they didn't know the weight the word biopsy carries. Saturday, Sunday, and Monday came and went, and we kept ourselves busy. Just like the picture from Florida, there is a picture of me from that weekend sitting on our pontoon wearing a black jacket and a light blue shirt and half-smiling. Underneath the jacket, I was still wrapping my chest with the Ace bandage and the weight of worry was still with me. In the photo, my hair is blowing and I am wearing sunglasses.

Tuesday was the 4th. On the evening of the 4th, Doug and the girls went to some friends' cabin to watch their fireworks' show, but I stayed back at the cabin and started cleaning. We were planning to head out in the morning, so I thought I would get started on the clean-up that comes after a weekend of festivities and also, I just didn't want to really be around people.

I am one of those people that love cleaning and find it relaxing and therapeutic. When I can put my external surroundings in place, my internal self is calmer. I am guessing I stayed up until they got back from the fireworks, but I don't really remember.

We were up fairly early with a plan to finish cleaning and then head home. We got "the call" at about nine in the morning. While the Nurse Navigator had promised a call in early afternoon, the pathologist who read the slides called Doug out of courtesy. She knew he was part of the health care community and wanted to deliver the news herself. When the number for Pathology Associates popped up on Doug's cell, he stepped outside the front door and paced around the yard as he talked. I followed him and watched him; it only took me seconds to realize the news wasn't good.

"Ok, so it is cancer. Darn it, we were so optimistic that it wouldn't be," I don't remember his exact words, but I remember that he said something like that. He talked for a few more minutes while I sat on the front steps, deflated.

"Okay, we will have the receptor status later today then?" he asked.

I am sure there was more to the conversation, but I don't remember that. I do remember that I was just wearing the t-shirt I had slept in and an oversized jacket of Doug's I had slipped on before I came outside. It was gray and a little bit cold for a July morning.

Eventually, we came inside and told the girls. We all sat on our big green sectional and cried. I don't think Doug did, but the girls and I did. The sky that had looked gray ten minutes before turned dark and the heavens unleashed sheets of rain. I watched the rain hit the lake in sheets and felt like, in the last ten minutes, my whole world had changed. I was still in Doug's oversized coat. My daughters sat around me crying, and I couldn't really comfort them. We held each other for a long time, and with the rain, it felt like the world was mourning with us.

But….. we couldn't stay in that place, on that sofa, forever. I had been hoping so deeply that the call would be different, that we would all just breathe a sigh of relief and be giddy with happiness. I had even pictured how the call would play out in my mind.

But the call wasn't good, and Doug had to work on Thursday and now we had an appointment with the surgeon early the next morning. Doug called his office and asked the scheduler to cancel his first appointments the next day so he could be at the surgeon's office with me. And so, I got up, and kept cleaning and packing. The girls helped, too, and by lunchtime we were on the road, sitting in Doug's truck, pulling the trailer with our bikes behind us. We had hardly eaten anything, and so we stopped on our way home to get some carryout at a deli in a town called Rhinelander, WI. All of a sudden, I felt worried about what I was eating.

"Doug, do you think it matters what I eat? Can I have chips, meat? Do you think certain foods will make the cancer grow more quickly? What about Diet Coke? Should I go gluten free? Dairy free?"

"Honey, just don't worry about that right now. Just get whatever you want. It's okay."

I still remember that I got a french dip sandwich. My oldest, Grace, took psychology in high school, and she shared an article with me about the way that our memories imprint during traumatic events. It is called "Flashbulb Memory". According to dictionary.apa.org, a flashbulb memory is a "vivid, enduring memory associated with a personally significant and emotional event, often including such details as where the individual was or what he or she was doing at the time of the event." That is how I remember that I didn't eat the bread. I got a fork when we picked up the food and just ate the beef out of the bun. The bun was already a little soggy anyway. I had to force myself to eat, and the food just sat in my stomach, heavy and unmoving.

FROM HOME TO MAYO AND BACK AGAIN

JOURNAL ENTRY BY HEIDI EDWARDS
JULY 14, 2017

Thankfully, my primary care doctor, Dr. Kane, had already set up an appointment with a breast surgeon, Dr. Soberg, at the initial visit (just in case). We were able to see Dr. Soberg at 7:30 a.m. the day after the diagnosis. She told us that I would most likely do chemotherapy followed by surgery followed by radiation. She was also able to secure an appointment at the Cancer Center THAT SAME AFTERNOON. The oncologist at the Cancer Center, Dr. Anand, agreed with her plan, but Doug and I felt like we needed to get a second opinion. Doug did his training at Mayo Clinic, and by the grace of God, we were able to be seen there the next day, Friday. We ended up being at Mayo on Friday, Monday, Tuesday, and Thursday. After an MRI, another ultrasound, another biopsy, a genetic consultation, and baring my affected breast to over 20 people, Mayo conferred with the treatment plan presented by the doctors at home.

Reflection

Like the phone call from the pathologist, the rest of that Wednesday, July 5th, and the entire rest of the week are vivid in my mind. The most important event on Wednesday, besides the diagnosis, involved Doug trying to get me seen at Mayo Clinic in Rochester, MN. We had lived in Rochester for three years while Doug did his ophthalmology residency. He called the Breast Clinic there and also made contact with two ophthalmologists he knew who practiced at Mayo hoping for an appointment as soon as possible. The pathologist from home also called us back on Wednesday letting us know that my receptor status was triple negative.

Also, Doug called my parents and told them the news. I couldn't do it because I knew I would start crying if I did. They told us they would come up the next day. I called other friends, though, and Grace made plans to go to a movie with some of her friends. I drove her to one of the friend's houses (the dad had offered to drive) and the mom came out to talk to me. I could tell she was sad for me because she got a little teary as we talked. I backed out of the driveway and started heading towards home. When I was about a mile from home, I completely broke down; I yelled and screamed and talked to God. I was scared and angry and full of despair. I told God that, and I know that he listened.

When Grace came home, she was equally wound up and worked up.

"Mom, my friends were laughing and joking and having fun. It's like they didn't even care. I am so sad, and I couldn't even focus. It was terrible. I wish I would have stayed home."

"Oh honey," I said, "They are only 14. They don't know what to say. They do care, you just can't expect too much of them because they don't know what to do or say."

But still, the pit in my stomach, the pit that I already had, got worse. I could feel it along with a feeling of nausea, shakiness, and weakness. I slept that night, though; all the anxiety of the day had exhausted me.

When I woke up, cancer flooded my brain. Sleep had been a respite; the waking was heartbreaking and getting out of bed and facing the day was even harder.

The morning brought a 7:30 a.m. visit to the surgeon. I was grateful to Dr. Kane for having the foresight to schedule an appointment with Dr. Soberg, the breast surgeon who handles a large share of the breast cancer surgery where we live. She was kind, direct, and empathetic, but very factual.

"With triple negative breast surgery, we almost always do neoadjuvant therapy. That means you will have chemo before surgery. That is because the prognosis for TNBC (triple negative breast cancer) is heavily dependent on the way the patient responds to chemo. By doing chemo first, we can tell if the cancer is responding to the chemo. Surgery will take place after chemo. With the information we have right now, you are probably a good candidate for a lumpectomy. Surgery would probably be followed up with radiation."

Even while I was sitting there, in her office, in yet another gown, I didn't feel like this was happening to me. It didn't seem real. I felt outside of myself, like I was a third person in the room observing all that was happening. Dr. Soberg asked us if we had an appointment at the Cancer Center set up yet.

"We are expecting a call from them this afternoon to set up an appointment," Doug said.

"Let me call over there and see what I can find out for you," she said.

As we were wrapping up our conversation with Dr. Soberg, Doug got a call from the Breast Center at Mayo Clinic, wondering if we would be able to come to an appointment the next day.

"What do you think, Heidi? Can we do it?"

"Yes," I said, "definitely!"

Mayo asked us to bring two things to the appointment the next day: the radiology images and the cell block. While we waited for Dr. Soberg, Doug called the radiology clinic and asked them to put the images on a CD and told them he would pick them up shortly. He also called the pathology clinic and requested to pick up the cell block. (The description below explains what a cell block is.) Basically, cells are "preserved" after the biopsy. That way, if more testing is needed, the pathologist (or another pathologist) can do more testing on the cells.

According to Canterbury Health Laboratories,

Cellular material is centrifuged into a concentrated cell pellet which is then made into a "clot" using the Thrombin clot method. The resulting clot is then fixed in Formalin for 15 minutes before transferring into a Histology tissue cassette. The clot is then processed through normal histology preparation steps to produce a "cell block". The cell block can then be cut into sections for microscopic examination or ancillary testing. e.g. immunocytochemistry/FISH.

The fact that we were able to get into Mayo was good news that was followed by more good news from Dr. Soberg.

"Actually, if you guys are able, Dr. Anand is willing to see you at 4:00 this afternoon," she said.

She was met with a grateful, "YES!" from both of us.

After thanking her, we left and Doug went to pick up what we needed for Mayo and then headed back to work. He called his office again to tell them he needed to be done around four and to tell them he would be gone on Friday.

I went home and probably did what I do every day—laundry, dishes, cooking, etc. I planned to meet Doug at the Cancer Center at 4:00 which meant I left the house at about 3:45 to head there.

I had driven by the Cancer Center tens of times, maybe even a few hundred times. Before this, almost every time I had driven past, I had felt a twinge of sadness for the cancer patients. I had imagined what it might be like to be a cancer patient. Prior to my diagnosis, I had had a few people close to me who were diagnosed with cancer. My father-in-law died of lung cancer when he was 52. The cancer started out in his lungs, and then metastasized to his brain. My best friend's dad died of kidney cancer literally days after we finished our freshman year of college. I knew that people got cancer, but I didn't know what it felt like to be diagnosed with cancer. I had imagined cancer to be like the song *Cancer* by My Chemical Romance where the image of cancer is pretty bleak. The song is from the perspective of a young man who is close to death. In the song, he is basically saying his goodbyes and preparing for his funeral. I didn't know it then, but not all cancer experiences are like the experience portrayed in the song. If you haven't heard it, it is a good listen, but get your tissue(s) ready, you might cry, especially if you have had a personal experience with cancer.

And so, when I entered the Cancer Center, I was angry and scared and surprised to be there and very, very scared of dying. I was very, very scared of suffering like the young man in the song and not ready to embrace or even accept a cancer diagnosis.

Before I met with my oncologist, I met with the radiation oncologist. Doug wasn't there yet, so I met with him myself and I was a sobbing mess.

Retrospectively, I don't think a visit with the radiation oncologist was necessary because:

I never ended up needing radiation.

Even if I had needed radiation, it wouldn't have been for about 7 months, at which point I would have remembered nothing about the visit.

From my own perspective, I think there are instances where people experience "information overload". I personally feel that, in times of crisis, information should be given on an "as needed" basis, doled out as needed. What I needed at that time was a clear explanation of my disease, the prognosis, and the immediate plan for addressing it. That said, I realize that I am only one person, and there are probably lots of patients who would have liked to meet with the radiation oncologist. Still though, what I needed most was the immediate plan.

Dr. Anand, my 5'5" (maybe) oncologist who was born outside the US helped with that.

Quite honestly, I would do anything in the world for that man-anything. I don't know where he trained, but I know there are thousands of folks in north central WI who are beyond grateful that a man who was born halfway around the world ended up in Wausau.

After I met with the radiation oncologist, I was escorted to another room at which point Doug arrived. We sat in this second exam room and clung to every single word Dr. Anand said. He did another physical exam and then told me I could come down from the exam table and sit next to Doug. He got a pen and started drawing and writing on the white paper. He started with triple negative breast cancer 101 and then moved on to the prognostic information.

My breast cancer education had begun.

Receptor Status:

According to Dr. Anand, one super important thing about breast cancer is receptor status. In a biopsy or during surgery, cells are taken out. One thing the pathologist looks for is whether or not the breast cancer cells have proteins that are estrogen or progesterone receptors. If they do have these proteins, when the hormones estrogen and/or progesterone attach to these proteins, the cancer is "fed" or "fueled". A third protein receptor that cells sometimes have is for the protein human epidermal growth factor receptor 2 (HER2). Some breast cancer is fed by estrogen, some by progesterone, and some by HER. Some breast cancer is fueled by all three and is called triple positive. Some breast cancer is fueled by none of these, as in my case, and is triple negative breast cancer. In the breast cancer world, there is always a reference to ER/PR/HER2 status. Patients will share their status like they are sharing the number of kids they have. Patients start their stories Stage 1, ER+/PR-/HER2+ or Stage 3, ER/PR-/HER2+ or Triple Negative or Triple Positive, etc.

Staging:

Based on the information we had at this point, Dr. Anand guessed my cancer was Stage One. That said, more imaging was needed to confirm or deny this.

Treatment:

He shared with me what he would recommend which was four cycles (two weeks apart) of a drug cocktail, adriamycin and cytoxan (AC). That combo would be followed up by 12 weeks (once weekly) of a drug called taxol (T). Once the chemo was complete and I had recovered sufficiently, I would be ready for surgery. Dr. Anand told me I would probably be a good candidate for a lumpectomy, but surgery was still a long way down the road. Whether or not I would need radiation depended on whether or not the cancer was in the lymph nodes and/or how the tumor responded to chemo. I started to understand that cancer follows an if/then pathway.

Prognosis:

This was probably the information that we cared most about.

I am sharing part of an article from The American Cancer Society's website cancer.org titled "Triple Negative Breast Cancer". The article begins by stating,

> Triple-negative breast cancer differs from other types of invasive breast cancer in that it grows and spreads faster, has limited treatment options, and a worse prognosis (outcome).

The article also shares five-year survival rates, which Doug and I were particularly interested in.

> Where do these numbers come from?

> The American Cancer Society relies on information from the SEER* database, maintained by the National Cancer Institute (NCI), to provide survival statistics for different types of cancer.

> The SEER database tracks 5-year relative survival rates for breast cancer in the United States, based on how far the cancer has spread. The SEER database, however, does not group cancers by AJCC TNM stages (stage 1, stage 2, stage 3, etc.). Instead, it groups cancers into localized, regional, and distant stages:

> Localized: There is no sign that the cancer has spread outside of the breast.

> Regional: The cancer has spread outside the breast to nearby structures or lymph nodes.

> Distant: The cancer has spread to distant parts of the body such as the lungs, liver or bones.

> 5-year relative survival rates for triple-negative breast cancer

Based on women diagnosed with triple-negative breast cancer between 2010 and 2016.

SEER Stage

5-year Relative Survival Rate

Localized	91%
Regional	65%
Distant	12%
All stages combined	77%

Understanding the numbers

Women now being diagnosed with triple negative breast cancer may have a better outlook than these numbers show. Treatments improve over time, and these numbers are based on women who were diagnosed and treated at least four to five years earlier.

These numbers apply only to the stage of the cancer when it is first diagnosed. They do not apply later on if the cancer grows, spreads, or comes back after treatment.

These numbers don't take everything into account. Survival rates are grouped based on how far the cancer has spread, but your age, overall health, how well the cancer responds to treatment, tumor grade, and other factors can also affect your outlook.

The citation for the entire article is in the Works Cited page.

Dr. Anand also shared that the prognosis for TNBC is heavily dependent on how the cancer responds to the chemo. For instance, even if the cancer is localized, but does not respond to chemo, the prognosis is poor because the cancer will grow. On the other hand, if the cancer is regional, but responds well to chemo, the prognosis is much better. That is why chemo is done quickly and that is why the response to chemo provides valuable prognostic information.

We told Dr. Anand that we were planning to head to Mayo Clinic the next day.

"That's fine," he said, "I think that they will probably tell you the same thing, but it will make you feel better."

We left together, and we felt just an ounce of relief. It wasn't much more than an ounce, but it was still an ounce.

I remember that we both felt very confident in Dr. Anand right from the beginning. We considered just skipping the whole Mayo visit because the more voices you bring into a situation, the more voices you have to listen to and the more confused you might get. It is easier to just listen to one voice. Plus, we were tired and traveling the four hours felt like a big effort. We have a dear friend, an OB-GYN, who had told us to go to Mayo in the first place.

We called him on the way home, and told him we were thinking of just bagging the trip to Rochester.

"Guys, you have to go. I am telling you in no uncertain terms that you have to go. It is worth your time and effort. Please, just go."

When we got home, my mom and dad were there, having just arrived from Iowa. My heart hurt for them, and I hated, just hated that they had to go through this with me. I tried not to let them see my worry, though, and tried to remain confident and upbeat for their sake.

Lou and Judy are tough cookies, though, as they have like most people who make it to their mid-seventies, seen a lot of heartache.

And so, we went to Mother Mayo. Doug had completed his ophthalmology residency at Mayo Clinic in Rochester, MN, and we had not been back since the day he finished. But, as children do in a time of crisis, we returned to a mother figure—a figurative mother in this case, a mother that seems wise and comforting, a mother that you can place your trust in, a mother that has stood the test of time. If you have never been to Mayo, it is something to behold, it is like a museum in its physical appearance, a tightly run business in its professionalism, and beyond comforting as a patient. (As I edit this a few months after writing it, I realize it sounds like a commercial, but the emotion and respect is still present.)

We made our way to Mayo the night before because our appointment was at eight in the morning. We didn't arrive in Rochester until late, probably around nine. The hotel we were in was clean enough, but really old and not very nice, and this added another layer of unpleasantness and sadness. For the first time in the last 36 hours, Doug broke down sobbing. This is a man I have only seen cry a handful of times in the almost 30 years we have known each other. We both felt the fear of what breast cancer might do to me, to him, to the girls, and to our family.

Our initial appointment was with an internist (someone trained in internal medicine) in the Breast Clinic who was kind of like the gatekeeper. Dr. Suta (also born outside the US) had a medical student with her, which is pretty much modus operandi at Mayo. We gave her the images and the tissue block. She decided what other tests and/or imaging were needed next, the most important next piece of information being a breast MRI. She made a few calls.

"Well, we can get you in for the MRI at about noon. Before you do that, though, I want you to go to the lab and get some blood work. I will see you back here at 4:00 and we can discuss the results of the MRI and what the plan will be going forward."

Getting blood work didn't bother me at all, but the breast MRI was just weird. As I was starting to realize, in breast imaging (and probably all imaging), there are different stations the patient passes through. Station One—change into a gown that opens in front. Station Two-get an IV in your arm (only for some imaging), Station Three-wait in the inside waiting area with all the other patients who are gowned and ready to go, Station Four—enter the actual MRI room. I am sharing some information from the American Cancer Society that explains the exam really well. The article is titled "Breast MRI".

MRI scans are usually done on an outpatient basis in a hospital or clinic. You'll lie face down on a narrow, flat table. Your breasts will hang down into an opening in the table so they can be scanned without being compressed. The technologist may use pillows to make you comfortable and help keep you from moving. The table then slides into a long, narrow tube.

The test is painless, but you have to lie still inside the narrow tube. You may be asked to hold your breath or keep very still during certain parts of the test. The machine may make loud, thumping, clicking, and whirring noises, much like the sound of a washing machine, as the magnet switches on and off. Some facilities give you earplugs or headphones to help block noise out during testing.

The most useful MRI exams for breast imaging use a contrast material called *gadolinium* that's injected into a vein in the arm before or during the exam, which helps to clearly show breast tissue details. (This is not the same as the contrast dye used in CT scans.) Let the technologist know if you have any kind of allergies or have had problems before with any contrast or dye used in imaging tests.

It's important to stay very still while the images are being made.

Again, the citation is included in the Works Cited page.

After the MRI, Doug and I went to get some lunch. This is my description-not Mayo's—but here goes—Mayo is the Disneyworld of health care. It is its own microcosm. Most of the Mayo campus is connected by tunnels (a subway) underground. This is very advantageous because Rochester is in Minnesota, and Minnesota is very cold in the winter. The tunnels are utilized by health care providers, staff, and patients. The subway level has candy shops, clothing shops, shoe shops, and gift shops mixed in with coffee shops and some quick service dining. There are also a few shops specific to health care needs. For example, there is a drug store, a post-mastectomy store, etc.

Where did we eat? I don't remember exactly, but it was Italian, and again, I struggled to get the food down. I do remember that we got a call while we were eating from the Breast Center asking if we could come now, about 2:30 p.m. instead of 4:00 p.m. I felt my breath get more shallow and I wondered what the call meant. I felt almost dizzy as we walked.

We arrived back at the 2nd Floor of the Gonda Building where I checked in and then I sat and then got up and then sat and then got up. Finally, we were called back. We had only been sitting for a little while when Dr. Suta walked in and shared the news.

"Well, Heidi, the MRI is a little bit concerning. We are seeing an area of concern that is larger than we initially thought, closer to 5 cm. It could be a hematoma from the biopsy, but we are not sure. We need to do at least another ultrasound to take a second look. Also, there are a few lymph nodes that are suspicious for cancer. We will need to biopsy those."

My heart sank and the blood rushed out of my face.

She went on, "We will work to get those tests scheduled for next week."

Doug, as he would until I was out of the woods, started advocating for me.

"I know the biopsy will have to wait, but is there ANY WAY we can do the ultrasound yet today? This will be just a terrible weekend if we think we are looking at a tumor that is three times bigger than what we originally thought. We already had a pretty shitty last weekend and this will be tortuous if we have to sit on this all weekend."

Dr. Suta looked pretty skeptical about the possibility of an ultrasound, but she picked up her phone and called radiology. By the grace of God, some kind and generous radiologist was willing to do the exam late on a Friday afternoon when I am sure her own spouse and kids were waiting for her. I promised myself never to begrudge Doug the chance to offer a patient comfort at night or on a weekend.

Soon, I was back at the Breast Imaging Center for the second time that day, back to the dressing room and the white gown, back to the inside waiting area. I found it almost impossible to be still or to stay composed. I pressed myself into the waiting room chair and moved my feet heel to toe, heel to toe, tried to take deep breaths, and imagined how the scene might play out. I took a warm blanket from the staff member who was, I am sure, glad that I was the last patient of the day. Finally, after nearly 30 minutes, a technician came and got me. This time, though, it was not the technician doing the exam. It was the radiologist herself. I looked at the grainy black and white screen as she worked, but I had no idea what I was looking for. When she was done, I asked her,

"Do you mind if my husband comes in to hear what you think?"

"Yes, I will call up to the waiting area and have him come back," she responded, not giving me any indication of whether her impressions were positive or negative.

She left for a while and returned with Doug following behind her.

When Doug entered the room, she started talking.

"Well, I think we can go with the first ultrasound and guess this tumor to be under two centimeters. I think what the MRI is picking up is the blood that collected around the tumor from the biopsy."

At that moment, we were elated, desperate for any piece of good news.

"We are still recommending the biopsy of the nodes, though. I just checked and we have you scheduled for that on Tuesday at 11:00 a.m. Also, Dr. Suta just called and let me know that she was able to get an appointment with the genetics counselor on Monday morning. When you come on Monday, you can check and see if there is any way they can do your biopsy that day so you don't have to stay another day. Before you leave, stop at the desk and they will give you a copy of your itinerary."

We did as she directed and we left feeling lighter. We celebrated by having dinner before we left, and I was able to eat for the first time in days.

We spent the weekend at home, but the joy and relief we had felt upon leaving was short-lived as we thought about the week ahead. Doug had to work the following week, but my Mom and Dad were able to stay. On Sunday night my Mom and I got back in the minivan and headed to Rochester. We stayed at the same hotel where Doug and I had stayed which just made the mood seem worse. There is just something about a dumpy hotel room that is kind of depressing. (I was a Mayo newbie and didn't realize that there were better options out there.)

Mom and I woke up in good time to meet with the genetics counselor. I don't think that having or not having a genetic mutation would have changed the course of chemo, but it would definitely change the surgical course. For example, if I turned out to be BRCA+, I would most likely want to have a bilateral mastectomy and perhaps an oophorectomy, removal of my ovaries.

Mom went with me to meet with the genetics counselor. The counselor asked lots and lots of questions and then sent me to the lab again for more blood. Mom and I had lunch in the subway level and then decided to find a different hotel for the night. We went back to the parking garage and drove to a different hotel that was probably about seven miles from Mayo. It was a bit better, but still kind of dumpy. I have always been very affected by my surroundings; the physical surroundings of a place seem to take on emotion for me, and I feel like I soak up the emotion. Maybe everyone is like that; I don't know.

The rest of the day was a blur, and I don't know what we did. I am sure Mom was keeping it together for me and I was keeping it together for her. I do remember an hour or so of deep distress when I just lost it in the hotel room; I sobbed and in the sobbing I released some of the agony. Tuesday morning brought the lymph node biopsies. We drove from the hotel to Mayo so that we could easily leave after the procedure, procedure being a catch-all word for a whole bunch of crappy things. Procedure seems like a clinical, cold word to me and that is appropriate.

When you go to Mayo, you are seen by a whole team of people: nurses, medical students, interns, residents, chief residents, fellows, and staff physicians because Mayo is a teaching hospital. The person doing my biopsy was a radiology resident. A radiology resident is someone who has completed medical school, but who is in their training to become a radiologist. As a rule, radiologists are the physicians who read and interpret the images from MRI, CT, x-rays and other imaging tests. However, there is also an area of radiology called interventional radiology; interventional radiologists use the images to locate the exact area of concern and obtain a biopsy. This is what occurred when I had the breast biopsy and now a radiologist was using the MRI images to locate the suspicious lymph nodes under my armpit. It took a fair bit of time while the resident worked under the attending (a doctor who is teaching) to get the samples. When they were done, I heard,

"We are all done. The samples will go to pathology. Dr. Suta will call you when we have the results. It might be this afternoon or it might be tomorrow morning."

I don't remember if we ate before we left. I know we made it to the car and I drove. The drive from Rochester to home was about four hours. I was OK for about the first two and a half hours and then I just started feeling considerably weaker and more anxious. I felt like I literally could not drive any more. So, I pulled over and asked my Mom to drive. I watched as she adjusted the mirrors and the seat and started driving. I put my head back against the headrest and closed my eyes, and then my cell phone rang....

"Hello, Heidi, this is Dr. Suta from Mayo. I just wanted to let you know that the samples came back negative, and we did not find any cancer. This does not 100% mean that there is no cancer, but it is a good sign. The last step is to have you meet with the whole team to decide on the best treatment plan for you. We don't have a time set for that yet, but we will call you soon to set it up."

"Thank you so much, Dr. Suta, you totally made my day, my week, my month. I am so relieved," I said.

Of course, my Mom, who was driving, was listening and she was jubilant as well. I called Doug and my dad, and I don't know who else. I could breathe again because each bit of good news was so good.

Mom still drove the rest of the way back. I was exhausted, and I am sure that she was too.

The next day we got yet another call from Mayo that the whole BREAST TEAM could meet with Doug and me on Thursday. We had a late morning appointment, so we got up early and drove there and back the same day. Again, as Mayo is a teaching hospital, we saw a lot of people besides the nurse, surgeon, oncologist, and radiation oncologist. I think we may have also visited with the plastic surgeon, med students, residents, and a social worker. My brain was so exhausted at the end of it all as I am sure that Doug's was, too.

As Dr. Anand had predicted, Mayo agreed with his recommendation of chemo first, followed by surgery, followed by radiation (possibly). They also agreed with the choice of drugs for chemo.

Chemotherapy is managed by an oncologist and she was the one who shared this news. However, I also met with the surgeon who told me that a lumpectomy would likely be possible, but that a mastectomy was also an option. Just as at home, the radiation oncologist who met with me told me that radiation may or may not be necessary. (As I mentioned earlier, I kind of wondered at the time and I still wonder now—why was it even necessary to get the radiation oncologist involved at this point. More doctors-more ideas-more confusion...... If I had been the one in charge, I would have just had the patient talk to the oncologist about the chemo because that was the first step in a long series of treatment. I think the same could be said for meeting with the general surgeon as my surgery did not occur for almost six months post-diagnosis. That said, I recognize that not everyone's brain works the same as mine does, and there are many people who likely want to speak to all the players on the team.) I also met briefly with the plastic surgeon, but again, it was just too much to process at the time. My mind was focused on the chemo.

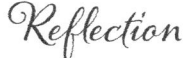

Reflection

My memories of this time are mostly connected to my own emotions. I acknowledge that my diagnosis affected all the people who love me very deeply-my husband, Doug, my daughters, Grace, Avery, and Lauren, my parents, Lou and Judy, and of course, my brothers, my extended family, and so many friends. Grace was just about to enter ninth grade when I was diagnosed, and Lauren and Avery were just about to enter sixth grade. In our district, sixth grade marks the beginning of middle school, and ninth grade marks the beginning of middle school.

Lauren and Avery were only eleven when I was diagnosed. They were at the precipice of big life changes themselves—moving from elementary to middle school and going from a class of about fifty to a class of about 350. They were starting middle school cross country and Avery was beginning her horsemanship journey. I am not sure what level of awareness they had about the seriousness of the diagnosis. About a year ago, I did find a journal entry that Avery wrote during this time for her English Language Arts class where she wrote about my diagnosis, my trips to Mayo and the Cancer Center, and about grandma and grandpa coming a lot.

Grace, on the other hand, was much more vulnerable at this time. My diagnosis seemed to trigger in her a great deal of anxiety and worry. She put some of this uncomfortable emotion and energy into cross country, but I was very worried about her for a lot of my year of active treatment and surgery. Worry about her added to my sense of grief and sadness.

Doug, well, Doug was a ROCK during this time—not an exaggeration. He threw himself into cancer research, particularly triple negative cancer research from the day of diagnosis. Even as we were driving home from Mayo, he was on the phone with the Cancer Center, asking when we could get chemo started. He had them on speaker phone as we headed east. The car already knew the way, having made three trips to Rochester in less than a week.

"I will be in contact with Dr. Anand," the woman on the phone said, "we will call you back tomorrow and let you know what the plan is." Even though we didn't arrive home until late, Mom and Dad went home to Iowa with a promise to return for the first chemo.

TREATMENT PLAN

JOURNAL ENTRY BY HEIDI EDWARDS
JULY 14, 2017

OK....so here's the plan. I will begin chemo on Monday here at home. I will do 4 cycles of Adriamycin and Cytoxan (I will refer to as AC in my writing going forward) that will be two weeks apart. After that, I will do 12 weekly treatments of Taxol. If everything goes according to plan (I'm prepared for ups and downs), I will finish chemo right after Thanksgiving. Four to six weeks later, I will have surgery. Surgery opens up more questions—-lumpectomy, mastectomy, bilateral mastectomy, reconstruction, no reconstruction? The good news is that I don't have to make any surgical or reconstruction decisions right now since chemo will be "Part One" of treatment. Also, the results of the genetic testing could inform the surgical decision which will also impact the reconstruction decision.

Reflection

On Friday, June 14th, the same day I wrote my first three journal entries on CaringBridge, we got a call from the Cancer Center with a "plan". Things felt a little better as we had direction and we knew what the next week would look like-kind of. The plan for Monday was:

Report to the Surgery Center for port placement at 6:30 a.m. Have nothing to eat or drink after midnight. Borrowing from the National Cancer Institute, "a port is a device used to draw blood and give treatments, including IV drugs, blood transfusions, or drugs such as chemotherapy and antibiotics. The port is placed under the skin, usually on the right side of the chest."

Get an echocardiogram which is an ultrasound of the heart. I needed to get an echocardiogram before starting on adriamycin-the A part of the

AC. Adriamycin can cause heart damage, so a baseline heart function test is needed.

Report to the Cancer Center for the first chemotherapy treatment. The nurse told me I would have blood work first, followed by lots of education, followed by chemo.

That left the rest of the weekend. I still felt just fine physically. I called my hairdresser on Friday as well and asked her if she could give me a short cut in anticipation of shaving my head. She graciously told me to come in on Saturday afternoon at the end of her day.

A TEMPORARY NEW HAIR-DO

JOURNAL ENTRY BY HEIDI EDWARDS
JULY 16, 2017

The oncologist who will be directing my care (the very encouraging physician named Dr. Anand) told me that I would lose my hair about two weeks after the first chemo treatment. Bearing that in mind, I called my amazing cosmetologist and asked her if she could squeeze me in for a short hair-cut. I figured it would be a way to begin the mental processing of my hair loss. When I arrived at the salon, a dear, dear, friend was also there. She has had long hair for the entire time I have known her. When I arrived at the salon, she was under the dryer and her hair was 10 inches shorter. Her words to me were, "You inspired me." This brought us all to tears-me, the cosmetologist, and Angela. I love my new cut, and I wish I could enjoy it longer than two weeks. I am going to get some hats, scarfs, and maybe a wig.

Reflection

Saturday, July 15th, was kind of a big day for the girls-it was the Wausau Chalkfest. This is an annual event in downtown Wausau where artists of all ages and skill levels create chalk art over a two-day period. Each artist is assigned an area of sidewalk to create a design of his or her choosing, but sometimes artists choose to create in teams as well. On Saturday, I spent most of the day at the Festival-with a break to go get my haircut. I saw lots of people I knew, and talking to people and hugging people brought lots of tears on my part. I remember feeling a little bit heartbroken and sad because I felt somehow separated from them. I felt......hmmmmmm...I don't know if punished/apart/alone are the right words, but something like that. Maybe there isn't a word in the English language for the emotion(s) I was feeling. I have spent a lot of time working as an English teacher, and I know that there are words that express emotion in one language that cannot be expressed clearly in another. There is an approximation, but not an exact equivalent. Maybe there is a word in another language.

Sunday brought the arrival of Lou and Judy again. Because Doug had to work on Monday, Judy was planning to be my chemo buddy. In a loving act that could only come from a Mom, she and my Dad had stopped at the Medford Outlet Mall as they traveled on Interstate 35N to pick me up a "first day of chemo" outfit. It was an Old Navy sweatshirt and some leggings. I found some humor in the purchase of a "first day of chemo" outfit, but at least I didn't have to worry about what to wear. Ha!

FIRST CHEMO AND WARNING— "DON'T LET THE DOG DRINK OUT OF THE TOILET"/ "DON'T WORRY IF YOU URINATE SHADES OF ORANGE/RED/YELLOW FOR A BIT"

JOURNAL ENTRY BY HEIDI EDWARDS
JULY 17, 2017

The day started at a local Surgery Center at 6:30 a.m. for port placement. I got a big hug from a former Eye Clinic employee (where Doug works) who is now working at the Surgery Center as the Chief Financial Officer. Doug, poor guy, left when they took me back and a nurse friend, Amy, was there when I came out to the procedure. She took me from the Surgery Center to another office for the heart echocardiogram where the tech told me my heart looked great and she wasn't used to working on such thin people. (That is sad because I still have a BMI of about 28.) She also told me I should consider cannabis oil for treating this cancer. Hmmmmmm.................... I told her I would think about that. From there Amy and I headed to the Cancer Center for treatment where my mom, sweet Judy, met us. While we waited to get the OK from the heart echo, I got the run-down on chemo. Big takeaways....Don't let the dog drink out of the toilet during chemo or it will be getting chemo as chemo drugs are excreted in urine. Don't worry if your urine is odd shades of red for a while. Drink a lot of water. Buy a wig if you want. (The Cancer Center has donated wigs if patients want, but I think Doug will spring for a new one.) The actual infusion did not take that long. You know it is powerful stuff, though, because the nurses administering it wear gloves and disposable gowns. Before I left, I got a Neulasta patch on my belly that will administer (with a small needle) the Neulasta to increase my white blood cell count 27 hours after chemo ends. And, Day One is done. Home to my Dougie and girls.

Reflection

Monday was a big day with three big events.

Port Placement—The breast surgeon I had met the week prior, Dr. Soberg, placed the port. Doug took me to the appointment, waited until they wheeled me back, and then headed to work. My friend, Amy, a nurse, was waiting for me when I woke up. After I was sufficiently recovered, she chauffeured me over to another building for an echocardiogram in her minivan. I am a huge fan of minivans, so I felt pretty much at home and also pretty blessed to have a nurse taking care of me.

Echocardiogram—My heart was A-OK to begin the chemotherapy and woo-hoo my BMI was only 28 (much to the tech's delight). That's a joke, kind of, as I think a healthy BMI is 24 or under. North-central WI, though, is not the healthiest place on the planet. We have LONG winters here, sometimes the better part of seven months. Beer is king and cheese is queen. Honestly, though, I love it here. I have lived here long enough that it is home; the twins were born here and Grace moved here when she was six months old. That said, the long winters and the cheese haven't done me any BMI favors. (I am not a beer drinker, but I LOVE cheese.) I have tried to lay off cheese a little bit post-cancer.

Chemotherapy—As the post above mentioned, the big event of the day was the first chemotherapy infusion. I don't remember if I had lab work or saw Dr. Anand before I went to the "treatment room", but I do remember being in the treatment room. It was a big open room with lots of hospital-like recliners in an oval shape. Shortly after I finished treatment, the Cancer Center did a big remodel with a fancy, schmancy treatment area, but I got cancer too early to enjoy that. Sometimes my timing is just a little bit behind-bad joke. Off of the large treatment room were two private rooms with hospital beds. The nurse asked me if I would like to receive my first transfusion in one of these rooms as they were open, which is not always the case.

"Sure, that would be nice," I said tentatively.

I sat in the room for quite a while because we had to wait for the cardiologist to read the echocardiogram. While we waited, the nurse did lots of chemo education for me. I learned lots of things that I reported above. One thing I did not note in my Caring Bridge post is that you shouldn't have sex for 72 hours after the AC chemo- just an FYI folks. A social worker also came in to talk to me, and the thing that I wanted to talk to her most about was my kiddos. She was great, but she didn't have a lot to offer in regards to this. Maybe this was because I was one of the younger patients. I did notice that most of the patients were older; they didn't look like they had sixth graders or ninth graders. Most of them looked like they had grandkids. As time went on, I learned a lot more about how to help and support my girls, but in those early days I felt really unsure. Amy stayed with me until my Dad dropped my Mom off. We all gabbed for a while, angel Amy left, and then Mom and I got the job done.

I felt OK when I got home, mostly just really tired. It wasn't until about nine at night when I started to feel nauseous. The way I felt for the next few days set the tone for the remaining three AC treatments. I had all my treatments on Mondays, and felt pretty decent until Monday night. Monday night I started to feel like I just got over a bad case of the stomach flu—weak and slightly pukey. This would continue until about Thursday with improvement each day from Monday night to Thursday. Then, I had about ten good days until I did it all over again.

NOT A BRCA CARRIER/CHEMO NAUSEA

Journal Entry by Heidi Edwards
July 19, 2017

I got the call from the genetics counselor at Mayo Clinic that I am not a BRCA carrier which is very relieving for me in terms of the girls and in terms of my brother and his children. The counselor unnerved me a bit when she said she was kind of surprised that I wasn't a carrier because of my age at diagnosis.

I did pretty well until about 9:30 on Monday night, and then a fair bit of nausea hit me. I haven't had this much nausea since I was pregnant with the twins. I tried the Compazine the doctor prescribed, but it didn't help too much. In the morning, we called the Cancer Center and they called in Zofran for me. Fortunately, the nausea subsided and I didn't need to use it. I was hoping I was home free, but last night was also difficult. The Zofran made things a bit better, but I think this just might be the dealio for a few days post chemo. I don't know...............

Papa and Grammy left on Thursday with a promise to return the night before my next treatment in about ten days.

WEEKEND BLESSINGS

JOURNAL ENTRY BY HEIDI EDWARDS
JULY 22, 2017

I made it through the first chemo, and felt reasonably normal by Thursday. By the time Friday (yesterday) rolled around, I could start counting my blessings.

Blessing One—I went for a walk up Rib Mountain with my dear friend (and our dogs) yesterday.

Blessing Two—Another friend stopped in on Friday and brought me an awesome gift bag that included a great hat that Lauren said was "the best we've seen". My friend also told me that she is organizing a small team for the upcoming Susan G. Komen race. Team Name—Hooters for Heidi!

Blessing Three—Yet another sweet friend, Helen, brought a delicious casserole for us for Friday night dinner. After dinner, Doug and I and the girls sat in the driveway and played with Ave's two guinea pigs, Max and Teddy. Every time Doug tried to move them from his lap, they cried and made their way right back.

Blessing Four—We were supposed to go on vacation this week, but in light of everything we cancelled the trip to Glacier. So, Doug is home this week, and we made the decision this morning to come up north for a bit and enjoy being here with each other.

I am still sad, and I am still scared, but I am also still so blessed.

BALD AND BEAUTIFUL?

JOURNAL ENTRY BY HEIDI EDWARDS
JULY 28, 2017

We knew hair loss was coming—we all knew—Doug, Grace, Avery, Lauren and I. While we were up North earlier this week, the subject came up while we were out boating and enjoying the perfect afternoon sun. (Lauren was working on perfecting her slalom skiing. She got up once, but summer will still offer her more opportunities for mastery.)

Once we started talking about hair loss, the conversation went something like this.

Ave—"Maybe you won't lose your hair."

Lauren-"She's gonna lose her hair, Ave, that's what the doctor told her."

Grace—"That is going to be so sad to just watch it fall out."

Me—"I think I will just call Hanna and have her shave it BEFORE it falls out."

Doug—"That's a good idea, Heid, why don't you do that."

My oncologist had told me that I would most likely start to lose clumps of hair around 13-14 days. So, last night, on the evening of Day 11, we did baldness on our terms.

After a nice, vigorous walk up and down Rib Mountain, we ended our day with a trip to our salon. We were basically the last folks there, and Hanna let Lauren and Ave cut some big chunks of my hair off. (Grace just couldn't.) Then, she shaved it, leaving just a bit of fuzz.

I thought I would cry, but I didn't. Ave cried when we got home. Everyone else had left the parked car, and she and I just sat in the front seat while she cried.

"Before, Mom, you didn't look different at all, but now people will be able to tell you have cancer."

She was right, and there was nothing I could really say, but a good cry did make it better.

WIGS 101

JOURNAL ENTRY BY HEIDI EDWARDS
JULY 30, 2017

On Saturday morning at 9:25, we found ourselves in the parking lot of a nondescript six story office building in St. Louis Park, MN.

Our destination—It's Still Me-a specialty wig shop for hair loss due to chemotherapy.

We made our way up the stairs to Suite 401. There was a small sign in the door that said, "In the Bathroom—Be Right Back". Like all the women on my mother's side of the family, I never miss an opportunity for a bathroom stop. (The twins compromised my bladder a bit as well.) Grace, though still young, never misses a bathroom opportunity, either.

Anyhow, when I returned to the office, we received a warm welcome from the owner of the store, Jan, who is also a breast cancer survivor.

She took us all to the back room and seated us around a large round table. She was just as interested in meeting us and hearing our story as she was in selling us a wig. She asked the girls how they were doing with everything and if they were feeling OK about my breast cancer.

After that, she started to tell us about the difference between synthetic wigs and wigs made from human hair. Here's the lowdown:

1. Synthetic wigs are much easier to care for, and hold their style much better.

2. Synthetic wigs are about a third the cost of wigs made from human hair.

3. Synthetic wigs are probably a better choice for low maintenance people as wigs made from human hair need to be styled and cared for a bit more.

My sweet Douglas was quick to tell me that I did not need to worry about the cost, but after hearing Jan mention the term "low maintenance", Grace spoke up.

"Mom, I think you're kind of a low maintenance kind of person."

I agreed completely, plus I am a budget minded gal. (I am my father's daughter.)

From there we learned about the different levels of quality in synthetic wigs.

Some wigs are only hand tied in the front. Some are hand tied halfway back, and some are fully hand tied. The benefit to hand tying is that it looks like you have a natural scalp. Higher quality wigs also have a more natural hairline in the front.

Even though I'm sure this wasn't terribly exciting for the girls, they listened attentively.

After our brief lesson, Jan got me in the chair and we started the fun part, trying on actual wigs. She was very skilled, and in about 20 minutes we had two wigs that were strong contenders.

The first looked very similar to the haircut I had before I was diagnosed. The second was similar but a bit longer. We sent a few texts with pictures out to my friend, Sarah, the most fashion savvy person I know, and decided to go with wig number one. We had saved a swatch of hair from Thursday's haircut, so we were able to use that to pick the right hair color.

Jan gifted me a special brush and stand for drying the wig after it is washed.

In addition to the wig, I also purchased some shampoo, conditioner and three hats.

Jan gave Lauren, Avery and I a little lesson on how to shampoo the wig.

Before we left, I got a picture with Jan, and she took a picture of the five of us.

As we thanked her, she shared with us that she feels very blessed to be alive. When she was diagnosed, her stepdaughters were just six and this year they graduated from high school. She also shared that the word that best sums up her emotions post-breast cancer is humbled. She is humbled to be alive, humbled to have a thriving business, and humbled to be able to help the women she serves. She is humbled that the Lord is using her in this way.

So, we came for a wig, and we left with a wig. (Actually, it will be shipped to my house by Wednesday.)

We left with more than a wig, though. Jan gifted us with hope, compassion, and the belief that we can find something beautiful in every experience.

CHEMO TWO DONE!!

JOURNAL ENTRY BY HEIDI EDWARDS
JULY 31, 2017

Just a quick update!!

I had my second round of chemo (the AC part) today. We arrived at about 9:45 a.m. and left at 2:30 p.m. There was lots of sitting around and waiting, so patience was key.

Fortunately, my dear friend Angela was there to take good notes for me and love me up.

I left with my Neulasta on board. It is a small device (on my stomach) that will automatically administer the Neulasta (to rebuild white blood cells) 27 hours after chemo is done. Then it can be taken off and discarded. Too bad it can't burn a little stomach fat while it's there! :)

Reflection

I remember that night after the chemo. When I came home, I went up to my bedroom to lay down for a little bit. (Louise came up and snuggled with me. She did that a lot after chemo. I wonder if she knew that I needed her. I wonder if she could smell the chemo in my body.) I was feeling a little sorry for myself; I remember that distinctly. I could hear Doug coming up the stairs and walking down the hallway. He opened the door and turned on the lights.

"Hey, Heid, you ready for a walk? Let's go to the quarry. The girls are going to come with."

"I don't know, honey, I just had chemo and I don't feel too well, maybe tomorrow."

"Nope, you need to get up and get moving. It will protect your heart and you will feel better. I promise," he said.

It took a little more coaxing, but within 15 minutes I found myself in the front seat of the minivan. Louise and the girls were also there.

"The Quarry" is an old granite quarry that has been transformed into an awesome hiking area. It is a reasonably steady, sweat inducing incline up to the top and the views are well worth the effort. Today, though, I was pretty dang proud of myself for any exercise I did and I was planning on about a 45 minute hike. Doug, though, had other ideas. He wanted to do about a four-mile-loop. About three miles in, I started to get angry at him.

"Doug, I just had some pretty bad chemo today. I think you are pushing a little bit hard. I am tired and dizzy and I feel like shit."

I don't remember my exact words, but I am sure it was something like that.

He wasn't upset; he was sympathetic and kind, and so were the girls. They gathered around me and supported me. One of the twins found me a nice walking stick. Doug grabbed one of my hands and G grabbed the other and we made it the last mile. Lauren gave me her water bottle and I took a big swig.

"I'm sorry, sweetie, if that was too much," he said when we made it to the car, "I just think it is really important to exercise right now. I think you need to exercise like your life depends on it."

I took that mantra to heart, I really did.

Our walks during chemo were very powerful medicine in many ways. In a practical sense, they protected my heart from the damage that AC can do. There is actually scientific evidence that supports this. Even more importantly, though, they were powerful emotional medicine. The walks reminded me that even though I had cancer in my BREAST, the rest of my body was HEALTHY AND CAPABLE AND STRONG. The walks reminded me that I was not sick. The walks gave Doug and I time to talk. Granted, we mostly talked about cancer, but that was OK. Doug literally MADE me walk even if I was not feeling like it, and that was exactly what I needed.

That day we walked at the quarry, but most of the time we "walked the hill" at a nearby state park called Rib Mountain State Park. The road leading up to the park ranger station is about a mile and a half and the change in elevation is about 600 feet, so it is a nice, steady climb and a three mile round trip hike. Climbing "the hill" became almost like a ritual from July to December. It was a way to take back the power and strength cancer took from me. There are about four big pieces of advice I would give to anyone dealing with cancer and one of them would be to EXERCISE as often as you are able and as intensely as you are able.

FISH PLANTERS AND FIFTEEN-YEAR-OLD HEROES

JOURNAL ENTRY BY HEIDI EDWARDS
AUGUST 6, 2017

It's Sunday night. Doug and I are snuggled up in our oversized chair. Louise is on the sofa, still recovering from her trip to the Pet Wash station (conveniently attached to a nearby car wash). The girls biked over to shower at the neighbors as our hot water heater went out on Friday. Doug is going to shower at work, and I will be OK until we get a new water heater tomorrow.

We had a good weekend. I have some amazing college friends that get together every summer, and this weekend happened to be our annual reunion. This year we were meeting in the Wisconsin Dells, a popular destination in Wisconsin, so I took off at about 4:00 p.m. Friday to meet the ladies (who had started their reunion on Thursday). Doug and the girls had planned to head up North which was a good thing in light of the hot water situation at our house.

I arrived to the shelter of the women who have known me for more years than they have not known me. We have been in and to each other's weddings, welcomed our babies together, and attended funerals for parents and siblings. We have visited each other's apartments and homes and communities. We have laughed and cried and rejoiced and agonized with each other. Once we moved past the initial hugs and greetings, we settled into the chairs on the patio of the condo we rented. Over pizza and snacks and wine, I told them the whole breast cancer story—from feeling the lump to finishing the second chemo.

We sat outside until the bugs started biting us and the air was too chilly for comfort. Once inside, they asked me to sit down and told me they had a surprise (or a few surprises). The first surprise was a huge fish planter. I had actually seen the planter at a little shop in Iowa last year during our reunion, but I hadn't gotten it. This year, when two of my friends were driving to the Dells, they stopped at the same shop where I had seen the planter, and bought it. The group of seven also gave me gift cards to some of my favorite restaurants. One of the ladies, Helen, had gotten everything ready for ten freezer meals they had prepared before I arrived. I had not cried at all on the patio, but the outpouring of generosity brought me to tears and soon we were all a heap of crying 44-year-olds, and one 45 year old.

Saturday was tranquil and "girlfriendy"—-breakfast, sitting by the pool, munching on snacks for lunch, and some outlet mall shopping. On Saturday evening we splurged at a nice restaurant, and near the end of the meal, a gentleman came over and got on his knees beside me.

"Can I ask? Are you in treatment for cancer?" he asked. (It was my "chemo" hat, of course.)

"Yes," I said. (In my mind, I thought he probably worked at the restaurant and was going to offer me a free meal.)

"My daughter just finished treatment for blood cancer in March. She has wanted to come over and give you a hug all night, but she was too shy, so I told her I would ask for her."

Before I stood up, he showed me a picture of her from March on his phone. She was perfect, and she was bald.

I got up and his daughter (sitting at a table close by) did, too. She told me she was 15 and she looked wonderful. Her hair had started to grow back. It was short, but I would have never known she had been in treatment so recently if I hadn't seen the picture. We hugged each other for a long time. Even writing about it now, my heart still aches with the pure connection I felt to this brave young woman. We both cried, and her dad did, too. Her dad told me that she had raised over $6,000.00 for cancer research.

"I just want to tell you to kick cancer in the butt," she said.

"I will," I told her. I told her about my girls and I told her she was beautiful and we hugged again.

Then, I sat down and she and her family left the restaurant.

I wish I had taken a picture with her, but I didn't think about asking. I am so grateful to her and her father for having the courage to reach out to me because it was a gift.

The whole weekend was a gift. Breast cancer sucks, chemo sucks, surgery will suck, and on and on, but this weekend I was gifted with friends and generosity and the courage of a 15-year-old girl and her dad. (I was also grateful to my husband for my time away.)

Reflection

I had been nervous before I arrived at the Dells to meet these "sisters". I didn't know how the time together would feel or how I would feel. When I stepped out of my minivan, I could feel my chest tighten a little and the anxiety creep in. I am trying to analyze as I write why I felt that way. Maybe it was because I was sad as this annual event that I looked forward to was affected by cancer. Maybe it was because it all felt so new and I was feeling fragile. Maybe it was because right now I was most comfortable at home and leaving felt scary. Maybe it was because I knew they would all view me a little differently or treat me a little differently.

The weekend (Friday night to Sunday morning) was good though. My suite sisters (we had all lived together in a suite during college) were so loving. The first night they gave me a room all to myself with a HUGE bed while four of them slept in the other room and two slept on a pull-out sofa. One of the suitemates had not felt well, and she left for the first night I was there just to make sure I would not get ill. Once she knew she was OK, she joined us again. Marcia, your kindness and self-sacrifice are still remembered. The second night, one of my BFF's, Jodi, slept with me.

I left with the back of my minivan full of stuff-the fish planter, the frozen meals, some gift cards, and some items I had picked up while shopping at the Outlet Center in the Dells. Three of us got matching gray Eddie Bauer dresses. I still have the dress and it is a keeper. The rest of the week was quiet. It was my OFF week, so no chemo-just normal life.

SUSAN G. KOMEN AND A VISIT FROM MY BROTHER, CORY

JOURNAL ENTRY BY HEIDI EDWARDS
AUGUST 13, 2017

We are all tired at our house, but it is a good tired.

The weekend started out with my brother's arrival on Friday evening. My younger brother, Cory, my sis-in-law, Jody, and their three kids, Katelyn, Brooklyn, and Braden, arrived at about 7. We enjoyed pizza brought to us by Heather from a local spot. We chatted and ate and all the kids (except G) hopped in and out of the hot tub. They stayed at a hotel, but before they left for the night my baby bro and I got a pic together—both of us bald. (All the cousins said I looked better bald than my brother, so that gave me a little boost—ha, ha, ha!) My brother and crew (minus Katelyn who stayed with us) stayed at a hotel and we all met back downtown at about 9:15 in the morning. We spent a great day together checking out Wausau, swimming at a local pool (not me), and going out for lunch. After grilling out at our house for dinner, they took off. Lauren and Avery were especially SAD to see their cousins go.

Sunday we were up early and met our team for the Susan G. Komen, Hooters for Heidi, in the Eye Clinic parking lot. Before we arrived, I was a bit worried that it would be a teary day for me, and I didn't put on any mascara. I don't usually wear mascara, so not really much change. As it turned out, not a tear was shed. I was moved by all the people who came to support not only me, but our family. My friend, Amy, is a mover and shaker and got the team going. (Thanks, Amy!) There were people there from my book club, from my neighborhood, special family friends, and friends we have gotten to know through the girls.

I walked, Grace ran with friends, Avery ran with Julia, and Doug ran/walked with Lauren.

I got a medal and some pink beads when I crossed the finish line. The woman who gave me the medal saw Doug with me and said, "Is this why you had to cancel my appointment in July?"

"Yep," Doug said, "I'm sorry."

"Well," she said, "I forgive you now. I'm a breast cancer survivor myself. I'll see you in September."

"Yes, you will," Doug responded.

"Good luck to you. If you ever need someone to talk to, tell your husband to get my number and give me a call," she said to me, adding a big hug to her offer.

We hung around for another hour or so, and then treated the younger members of the team to smoothies downtown at a fun coffee shop called the Paisley Mug.

We stopped for a quick grocery run while the girls hung out in the car.

Doug and I were done, but the girls had enough energy to do a one-mile color run at Wausau West.

We dropped them off, ran home to drop off the groceries, and then Doug ran back to get our girls.

Chemo is on the agenda for tomorrow, so now we are going to DO AS LITTLE AS POSSIBLE and just relish Sunday night. My Mom and one of my BFF's Jodi, will be arriving later tonight for chemo support.

Thank you to my brother and family and all the Hooters for Heidi folks for all the love this weekend.

ARE THESE ANGELS FROM HEAVEN?
NO, THEY'RE FROM IOWA!

JOURNAL ENTRY BY HEIDI EDWARDS
AUGUST 14, 2017

Both Doug and I grew up in Iowa. Granted, we have not lived there since 1999, but once we enter the state (from any direction) there is this part of us that just settles in because we are HOME.

We are all IOWA HAWKEYE supporters, even the girls. Iowa also has another college team, the IOWA STATE CYCLONES. My brother went to Iowa State, so we have some good, fun rivalry there. We relish Iowa sweet corn in late July, and the girls love catching fireflies in the summer. (Where are the fireflies in Wisconsin?) When we drive through Iowa we are amazed by the vast fields of corn and more recently, windmills. Like the citizens of our adopted state, Wisconsin, Iowans are salt of the earth people. They are hardworking, giving, and community minded.

So, when I needed some angels to come and hang out with me and the girls this week, calling on a few beautiful ladies from IOWA seemed like an OBVIOUS choice.

Last night, my dear friend, Jodi, and my Mom, Judy, arrived before dinner. My mom brought heirloom tomatoes and peppers from her garden and gifts from Iowa friends and Jodi brought stamping supplies for some crafting magic. Lauren and Avery love, love, love crafting.

This morning, Jodi went with me to the Cancer Center where I had a blood draw, saw my oncologist (who is very happy with the tumor shrinkage), and did chemo. My mom stayed with the girls (G had practice) and they did some cooking. My mom (and dad) have been AMAZING through this whole journey. (Dad stayed back this trip as he is the mayor of his small community and tonight is town council.) So, it was the two angels from Iowa, having traveled on I-35, I-90/94, and I-29, who came up to Wausau and stood in the gap for me.

And, like women have done for other women for centuries, they embraced me and saw what needed to be done and did it. They might not be angels, but they are God's daughters being used by Him. Or.........
maybe they are angels.

Reflection

As I reflect on my summer of 2017 (and the whole year that I was in active treatment for breast cancer), I again think about a piece my friend Helen shared with me (and the suitemates) in August of 2017. She shared this in an email shortly after we had all been together in the Dells.

Find Your Elephant Tribe
by Nichole Nordeman and Jen Hatmaker

In the wild, when a mama elephant is giving birth, all the other female elephants in the herd back around her in formation. They close ranks so that the delivering mama cannot even be seen in the middle. They stomp and kick up dirt and soil to throw attackers off the scent and basically act like a pack of badasses.

They surround the mama and incoming baby in protection, sending a clear signal to predators that if they want to attack their friend while she is vulnerable, they'll have to get through 40 tons of female aggression first.

When the baby elephant is delivered, the sister elephants do two things: they kick sand or dirt over the newborn to protect its fragile skin from the sun, and then they all start trumpeting, a female celebration of new life, of sisterhood, of something beautiful being born in a harsh, wild world despite enemies and attackers and predators and odds.

Scientists tell us this: They normally take this formation in only two cases – under attack by predators like lions, or during the birth of a new elephant.

This is what we do, girls. When our sisters are vulnerable, when they are giving birth to new life, new ideas, new ministries, new spaces, when they are under attack, when they need their people to surround them so they can create, deliver, heal, recover…we get in formation. We close ranks and literally have each others' backs. You want to mess with our sis? Come through us first. Good luck.

And when delivery comes, when new life makes its entrance, when healing finally begins, when the night has passed and our sister is ready to rise back up, we sound our trumpets because we saw it through together. We celebrate! We cheer! We raise our glasses and give thanks.

During this season of my life, I was the elephant in the middle. And that was both heartbreaking and heart-sustaining, but mostly heart-sustaining. It was heartbreaking because nobody really wants to be in a place where they need to be supported. However, it was mostly heart and spirit sustaining. It was only the love and support of family and friends and THE LORD that sustained me.

Maybe this is the time to speak to the fact that I do not think my situation is/was unique in its hardship. Many face struggles much, much more difficult than this. I am keenly aware of this. I think of people who receive terminal diagnoses or parents who care for children with terminal diagnoses. I think of parents whose children struggle with devastating drug or alcohol addiction or severe mental illness. I think of men and women whose lives are upended by an unexpected divorce or a job loss. The list goes on and on. My suffering is/was not unique or special. Still, though, it was traumatic and life-changing like all trauma is. So why am I writing this?

Writing is a way to process and put experiences to rest.

Writing is a way to reach others who have had, are having, or will have a similar experience and form a connection.

Writing is an art form, part of what makes us human.

OK, enough said on this. More on suffering at a later time.

·

TWENTY-FIVE PERCENT OF THE WAY THROUGH CHEMO......

JOURNAL ENTRY BY HEIDI EDWARDS
AUGUST 20, 2017

My friend, Keri, sent me a quote via text from C.S. Lewis........

> Imagine yourself as a living house. At first, perhaps you can understand what He is doing. He is getting the drains right and stopping the leaks in the roof and so on: you knew that those jobs needed doing and so you are not surprised. But presently He starts knocking the house about in a way that hurts abominably and does not seem to make any sense. What on earth is He up to? The explanation is that He is building quite a different house from the one you thought of-throwing out a new wing here, putting on an extra floor there, running up towers, making courtyards. You thought you were being made into a decent little cottage: but He is building a palace. He intends to come and live in it Himself. (Thank you, Mr. Lewis!)

I think this week it hit me that this is going to be a long journey and that my "house" was being knocked about in a way that hurt quite a lot and in a way it was hard to make sense of. I finished my third of four A/C (Adriamycin and Cytoxan) treatments. After the last on the 28th, I will have two weeks off before I begin 12 weeks of Taxol. I will receive infusions each Monday. Once that is done, we will move towards surgery 4-6 weeks later, possibly followed by radiation. The physical effects of chemo are becoming more pronounced, and a cancer diagnosis is an emotional roller-coaster.

Echoing Mr. Lewis yet again, all this "just seems to hurt abominably and does not seem to make any sense". From a certain perspective, it cannot and does not make sense for ANYONE, not just me, to struggle with serious illness. I know that many are suffering and have suffered much more than I have, and there is the question of whether there is any purpose in suffering.

I have decided to choose the perspective Mr. Lewis finishes the quote with, the perspective that God is transforming me. I am not sure that I will claim that God is transforming me into a palace, but maybe something between a cottage and a palace—a nice ranch or a classic two-story Colonial. I have to believe that I will be a different person as a result of this experience, that God will use this journey to transform me for His purpose.

On a lighter note, we had a good weekend. Doug and the girls did a SCUBA class all weekend. It started Friday night and was all-day both Saturday and Sunday. It was a BIG COMMITMENT, and they all PASSED!! I was supposed to take the class, but I decided to skip it and enjoyed a weekend of CLEANING and ORGANIZING. It was calming and therapeutic—there is just something about bringing order to the external that brings order to the internal.

Reflection

Re-reading this post made me think more about suffering and particularly about "suffering well"—a phrase coined by an amazing couple, Jay and Katherine Wolf. I recently became aware of their story through social media. According to an article by Leach Marie Ann Klett, titled "Stroke Survivor Katherine Wolf on Finding God in Suffering: 'There's Hidden Treasure in Darkness' ", Katherine was just 26 years old when she had a brain stem stroke that caused a brain bleed. Although she survived the 16 hour brain surgery, the new mother could not not talk, walk or swallow. She was also left with right-side paralysis, deafness in her right ear and double vision.

Klett goes on to share how, instead of living a life marked by self-pity and sorrow, Katherine and her husband, Jay, went on to make their mess their message. They both speak a great deal about what it means to suffer well. Katherine's husband, Jay, spoke about this in Klett's article. "Suffering well begins with not being so scared of the hard stories and really wrestling with the sad and bittersweet nature of life and not being afraid to talk about that and again find God in the midst of it. We don't need to be afraid of suffering because as believers, we can be confident that struggles will give us depth and a richness to our experiences with God and with one another."

I have thought a lot about what Jay said. Don't get me wrong, no one chooses to suffer. I cannot explain the suffering of parents who lose a child or children who lose a parent or the suffering that comes from divorce or from a slow debilitating disease and on and on. I know that my suffering was miniscule in comparison to the amount of suffering some have had to endure. Suffering is something no person would sign up for, but still, people suffer. Jay's idea of "suffering well" and what he says about the fact that our struggles give a "depth and a richness to our experiences with God and with one another" are ideas I had never really grappled with or considered as deeply as I did during my cancer journey.

JUST ENJOYING LIFE

JOURNAL ENTRY BY HEIDI EDWARDS
AUGUST 27, 2017

There is this feeling, when you are diagnosed with cancer, that you can start living again when you are done with treatment, whatever treatment might mean—-chemo, surgery, radiation—all of these, two of these, or maybe just one of these things. I have been tempted to fall into that trap, and even have, at times, given into the false belief that I cannot enjoy experiences because I have cancer. BUT, I know that is a defeating attitude. The whole reason I am doing treatment is to HAVE MORE TIME and EXPERIENCES and this week gave me TIME and EXPERIENCES.

So here are some of the many experiences I was happy to have this week..........

1. I was able to watch Grace run her first high school cross coun-try meet. Lauren and Avery and I drove up to Rhinelander, Wisconsin, on Thursday morning. It was a chilly morning, but the sun was shining and it was just thrilling to watch the high school athletes put themselves out there and compete. Grace did a great job, finishing 30th out of 135 runners.

2. I was able to see Lauren and Avery follow in their sister's footsteps and start middle school cross country practice. They didn't seem any worse for the wear each day after practice. The first night they were only home for about fifteen minutes before asking, "Can we see if Charlotte and Soph (their neighborhood buddies since birth) can come over?"
That said, by the end of the week, they were pretty tired. Grace snapped a pic of them, sent it in the family group chat, and captioned it—"Cross Country-End of Week One".

3. I was able to take all the girls to get before school haircuts. Avery decided to get short bangs cut, and the other two just got trims. Being bald, I didn't need a haircut, so I saved some money. :) I am already excited, though, about having hair again. Kay, I have loved your hair for years, and I am thinking of something along the lines of your gorgeous look when my hair grows back.

4. I was able to spend a great day with the girls on Saturday. We hit the Farmer's Market downtown, and then met Doug for lunch. (He was on-call and had a Saturday morning clinic.) Then, the girls and I went to the mall and all of us found a pair of shoes on the clearance rack at Younkers. (Editing Note—The Mall in our town has since been torn down.)

5. I was able to have dinner with some good friends and coffee with my Book Club.

6. I was able to hold a three-week-old baby and play a bit with his precious two-year-old sister.

7. My friend, Angie, sent me a beautiful PINK Coach leather wristlet. I was blown away by her kindness and generosity.... and fashion sense. I was thankful for the experience of owning my first Coach accessory.

I wasn't the only one who did some cool things this week......

Because I cannot do any manis or pedis during chemo, and because the girls were DYING to get pedicures with Doug, he caved and they all went for pedicures this afternoon. He really is a good, good father. This is his first ever pedicure. Only a real man would get pedicures with his daughters. (He also took them to Ulta before.)

I thank God for all these moments this week.

DONE WITH A/C

JOURNAL ENTRY BY HEIDI EDWARDS
AUGUST 28, 2017

Today I had my fourth and final treatment with Adriamycin and Cytoxan. Starting on September 11th, I will begin 12 weekly treatments of Taxol. Most women (and men) find Taxol easier to tolerate, so I am very happy to have completed this first milestone!

In lieu of using the word chemotherapy, I have consciously decided to use the word treatment.

It just sounds less anxiety provoking and more positive. (Maybe that's my linguistics background coming into play.) I have my Masters in Teaching English as a Second Language/Applied Linguistics.

The whole AC treatment day is pretty routine to me now and more predictable. Each day when I arrive, I check in and get a hospital band around my wrist with a unique barcode. In the lobby, the lab calls me and they access my port to do a blood draw and prepare for treatment. The port is just below my right collarbone. It is just under my skin and there are three dots that are very palpable. The nurse uses the dots as a guide to "access the port" with a needle. It is just one sharp prick, the needle is inserted and the port is open. The blood is drawn, and it is taken to the lab to make sure my blood counts are acceptable for treatment.

From there, it is back to the lobby. Today I positioned myself strategically away from a woman (accompanying her husband) I saw at another treatment who talked A LOT and told me "I was lucky that I only had to do chemo for five months". She's probably right, but I still found a nice spot on the other side of the room.

I was just starting on a book I found on a bookshelf in the lobby on "parenting during cancer" when I heard my name and the routine began. The chemo routine follows a very predictable pattern.

The CNA weighs me on the biggest scale I have ever seen. (It can be used for folks in wheelchairs.) I don't even look to see what I weigh. From there, I walk to an exam room to see a nurse who asks me the same questions every time. A brief bit later, my wonderful oncologist comes in and inquires, "How are you doing?" He is calm, and not in a hurry and we chat. We discuss Doug (Doug e-mails the poor guy on a regular basis with questions and studies and academic articles), and talk about the side effects of the next drug in my treatment plan, Taxol. Then, he does a physical exam. He cannot feel the tumor at all, and tells me that bodes very well for me. It is hopeful news, and I am relieved.

From there, I head to the infusion room. The infusion room at the Cancer Center is one large room with lots of hospital type recliners. I can choose any one I want, so I choose one on the end and by the bathroom (always good to be by the bathroom). It takes just a bit before a nurse is able to start, but a kind medical assistant brings me a pillow and warm blanket. After about fifteen minutes, the RN starts the anti-nausea drugs, a steroid, and a med called Aloxi. Once that is done, she starts the Cytoxan. It normally takes about 20 minutes, but this time the nurse slowed it down to take about 30 minutes. Sometimes, this drug can cause a burning in the nose similar to the burning one can get when water goes up your nose in a swimming pool—like chlorine in your nose. This happened last time, so we decided to run the med at a slower pace.

When that drug is finished, the I.V. starts to beep and the next drug is administered. The next drug is Adriamycin. It comes in two large vials and is red. The drug does not go through the I.V. Instead, the nurse directly pushes it slowly into the port. This drug has been dubbed the "red devil" by breast cancer patients. The nickname is well-deserved.

Once that is finished, it's time for the Neulasta patch and I'm good to go.

Reflection

I don't want to forget to mention that my dad was there with me during that treatment today. My mom was at home with the girls and they made homemade applesauce. Gosh, what would I have done without my parents? Of course, we would have survived. We would have had a messier house, gotten more carry-out, and asked the girls for more help I suppose. The point is, we were lucky because we had them to help out. The structure and rhythm of our family was able to remain pretty stable during treatment.

As I moved through treatment, it became less anxiety-provoking and more comforting because I KNEW WHAT TO EXPECT. I realize that so much anxiety and frustration in life, regardless of the situation, comes when people don't know that to expect. This awareness has helped me as a teacher and as a parent and as an advocate for others moving through a cancer journey.

A FEW LITTLE BUMPS, BUT ONWARD!

Journal Entry by Heidi Edwards
September 7, 2017

We spent the last few days before school started Up North. We were looking forward to enjoying a bit of sunshine and togetherness (and we did), but poor Doug had a nasty bout of gout. (That was the first little bump of the week.) He has struggled with this in the past, and we believe his recent rapid weight loss brought on this "attack". Poor fellow spent most of the long weekend icing his ankle and keeping it elevated. We did manage to sort of close up the cabin in the event that we don't get up there before the weather turns inhospitable and the lakes freeze over.

On Tuesday, my babies started school. It was a milestone as G started high school, and Lauren and Avery started middle school. They were up before their alarms went off on Tuesday, but today (Thursday) was a different story. Lauren was literally laying on top of her cell phone as the alarm was going off, and it did not wake her.

Lauren and Avery also had their first cross country meet on the first day of school. I'll be honest, I was a little nervous for those pumpkins. They went on a "loosening up" run on Labor Day and it was pretty rough. (I walked with them.) I am pretty sure I could have maintained their pace and I AM GOING THROUGH TREATMENT. That said, they proved me wrong on Tuesday and finished respectably. I was very proud of them.

Wednesday brought the second little bump of the week. My oncologist (partly at our request), scheduled a mammogram and ultrasound to see how things were progressing as I have completed the first round of treatment. So, I headed into the Breast Center at about 12:15 p.m. and had the mammogram first. It was kind of hard emotionally, but I made it through. Then it was back to the waiting room while I waited to be called for the ultrasound. A kind technician chatted with me as she got the images she needed, using the clip placed during the biopsy. The clip marks the place of the lesion. When she was finished, she left me in the room, still laying on the ultrasound table and told me the radiologist would come back and talk to me in 10 to 15 minutes. I honestly wasn't expecting that; I expected to just get the results from the oncologist at next Monday's appointment.

It was a long wait- long enough that I had to get up and leave to use the bathroom. I was thinking about all the things I wanted to do before I had to pick the girls up from school when the radiologist came into the room.

"Well," the doctor said, "The tumor looks about the same as it did when you had the first mammogram. Is that good news?"

My heart just dropped.

"No, it's actually terrible news. I don't know if you know this, but my prognosis is heavily based on how I respond to chemo. This just doesn't make sense because we can't even feel the lesion anymore. It is not good news if it's just the same."

At that, the radiologist brought me over to the screen and started showing me the images and measuring them, but I didn't really hear a word.

I started crying, and the physician just kept talking and talking and talking. I finally told the poor soul it was fine to leave and I would just talk to my oncologist soon.

Before the doctor left though, he/she said, "Don't worry, they're doing lots of amazing things with breast cancer these days."

I didn't respond, but I wanted to say, "I know, I'm doing them."

I left the room as quickly as I could, went to the changing room, sprayed on the deodorant they provide, and walked out to my car. Once in my car, I thought about texting Doug, but figured there was no point in getting him worked up when he still had a good three hours of work left to go.

Instead, I drove home, ate lunch, and folded some laundry. Right before I was ready to leave to go get Grace (who needed a ride to an offsite cross country practice), Doug called.

"How did it go babe?"

And then I completely lost it. I told him what the radiologist had told me. I told him it was a terrible idea to get a mammogram and ultrasound. I told him I was mad I had wasted my whole afternoon for nothing. I sobbed into the phone.

He told me he doubted what the radiologist had said, and told me he would call the oncologist. And that boy, my hero, did just that. He also told me that he was going to skip the evening meeting he had and come home.

"No, Doug, it's fine, it's really fine. I want you to go to your meeting."

He did go to his meeting and I calmed down and decided to wait until I heard from the oncologist because his opinion was really the only opinion that mattered.

At about seven, Lauren got a call from Doug.

"Hey honey," he said, "can you put your mom on the phone?"

"Great news, Heidi! Your doctor called me during the meeting and told me that the lesion has indeed shrunk considerably. Also, it is so much less dense that it is almost transparent in some spots. It looks like it has responded very, very well to chemo and is very chemo sensitive."

I am so grateful to the oncologist for taking the time to look at the images and call us and reassure us.

As it turns out, the radiologist just didn't have much familiarity with what he/she was looking at. I am not angry, but it was a very emotional day. I know the provider did not do anything wrong, so the point of my story is not to direct anger.

What is the point of my story?

I guess just to share my experience. Nothing more, nothing less.

In the end, all's well that ends well. Thank God that things are going well.

I also want to thank all the wonderful people in my life who have supported me with phone calls, texts, cards, meals, gifts, and prayers. I am absolutely overwhelmed with gratitude.

Reflection

One thing that we learned going through treatment was that when you are going through cancer treatment, there are lots of competing voices, lots of white noise, lots of opinions and ideas. These come not only from friends and family and the Internet, but also from health care providers.

Some of the competing voices/conflicting opinions I dealt with during my cancer trip were:

Port or no port—Our local Cancer Center uses a port for chemo, but Mayo does not.

Receptor status of tumor—Our local pathologists called my cancer a true triple negative; initially Mayo found my tumor to be 1-10% estrogen positive. (never 100% sure)

Lumpectomy or bilateral mastectomy-My docs locally really advocated for a lumpectomy, while the docs at Mayo stayed pretty neutral on that topic.

Need for more chemo after surgery- I ended up doing 24 more weeks of an oral chemo called Xeloda after my bilateral mastectomy. My oncologist at Mayo did not feel that was necessary, but my oncologist locally really recommended that additional layer of protection against recurrence.

Best method for reconstruction—I ended up using tissue expanders and implants for my reconstruction. Other folks are strong advocates of other methods.

Use of alternative options—Neither Mayo nor my local team advocated for the use of alternative treatments, but they did not discourage it either. I did add a number of other medications to my treatment regimen. (more on that later)

How does a girl (or guy) sort through navigating a cancer diagnosis (or any serious medical diagnosis)? I don't have the right answer, but I have a few suggestions:

Yes, a second (or third) opinion is good, but things start getting tricky when you get a fourth, fifth, and sixth opinion. At least for me, that is too many opinions and it is hard to keep track of all that you are hearing. At a certain point, you just have to make a decision based on the information you have.

Disclaimer: My cancer diagnosis/medical diagnosis was not that uncommon. I am sure that for people facing a rare cancer or medical diagnosis, getting multiple opinions is very important and may be the way the patient/family member finally discovers what is going on.

Secondly, find a person or a couple of people that you really trust. These are people (doctors) who are knowledgeable about your diagnosis and people who know YOU.

Next, there is a fair bit of "trusting your gut" in cancer treatment or any serious health situation. You have to trust yourself. You have to trust that you have done your research and made the decision that is best for you.

Finally, once you have made your decision or decisions, don't second guess yourself.

EVEN IF YOU HAVE BREAST CANCER, YOUR KIDS STILL.....................

JOURNAL ENTRY BY HEIDI EDWARDS
SEPTEMBER 12, 2017

It's 12:26 a.m. on Tuesday morning, and I can't sleep. I had my first Taxol treatment Monday afternoon, and I had a good dose of steroids to go along with it. Maybe that is the reason for my insomnia. While I was trying to nod off, my mind was composing this post, so I decided to just get up and type. I am wearing the orange-colored glasses Doug bought in bulk so that the light of the computer doesn't disturb my sleep. (If anyone needs a pair, we have A LOT of extra pairs in the laundry room cupboard.) I probably don't have to be too worried about sleep disruption from blue light BECAUSE IT IS PAST MIDNIGHT AND I AM STILL AWAKE, but I need all the help I can get.

I think part of the reason for my insomnia is my worry for my kiddos. Because, even if you have breast cancer, your kids still..........

1. Get colds that turn into bronchitis. (creds to Ave for that one) She has been hacking around the house while I keep reminding her to "cover her cough". Still, I worry about her because she has a bit of asthma/reactive airway disease. She and Lauren used a nebulizer daily from the time they were one to about age five.

2. Hurt their pinkie toe playing "Ghost in the Graveyard" at a birthday party. Our sweet podiatrist friend came over and examined her toe tonight and told us we should probably get it x-rayed. I will do that when Urgent Care opens in the a.m. (creds to Grace for that one)

3. Tell you they are not sure they like middle school after all. (creds to Lauren for that one)

Some of my child angst isn't from worry; it is just the plain pure fact that you can't stop being a mother just because you have cancer. Even if you have breast cancer, your kids still......................

1. Need three "1/2 binders" for school as soon as possible. (creds to Lauren)
2. Wonder if you can clean out the guinea pig cage because life is really busy for her. (creds to Ave)
3. Beg you to get the gum out of a favorite pair of Nike leggings with Goo B Gone because she needs them tomorrow. They are her favorite pair. (creds to Lauren)
4. Need to go to the orthodontist, need a fruit salad for a cross country team dinner, and need face cream. (creds to G, but actual real needs)
5. Wonder if now is a good time to buy a horse. (creds to Ave)

I have heard a few funny stories from other survivors. I read a blip from one woman who wrote about being in the treatment room, receiving chemo, and having her teen son call her and complain because there was no gas in the car. Another woman, after completing six months of chemo and surgery, was talking to her daughter about her daughter's upcoming tooth extraction. Apparently, her daughter was very scared and said, "Mom, have you ever had to deal with a serious illness?" The woman said, "Well, the cancer thing was pretty scary."

On Labor Day, Lauren was complaining about running and told me I needed to try to do something as physically hard as cross country. "Lauren," I replied, "will six months of chemo, a bilateral mastectomy, and possibly radiation count?" That gave her pause, but she still thought maybe cross country was harder.

At the end of the day, though, your kids (and your spouse) are what keep you going. They pull you out of yourself and make you keep moving forward. They keep you from making your identity a "cancer patient". Even though my post is a bit one-sided, the girls have been very loving and supportive and interested in this journey. They pray for me, love me, make me laugh, and make me cry.

On a side note, today's treatment went well, and I got through with no strange reactions. My sweet friend A was with me, and my Mom and Dad came up again to see how this treatment goes. Still blessed, still a mom, still real life.............

Reflection

Having kids and having cancer are a whole other topic. I could write a book on that honestly. In fact, there was a book I picked up in the cancer center lobby called "How to Help Children Through a Parent's Serious Illness". I actually had it in my car for the whole year I was going through treatment. There was one chapter about how to help children when you or your spouse has a terminal diagnosis. I glanced at that chapter and even read it. I did, at times, convince myself that I would not survive this cancer, and I felt (on a very small scale) what that felt like. I imagined not being there for high school graduations, or weddings, first jobs, first babies, etc. It is unimaginable and gut wrenching.

From the book, I learned that while there is no perfect way to navigate parenting and dealing with a serious health issue. However, ignoring it or not being honest with kids is the worst (and least helpful) approach.

My girls never went to chemo with me. The twins did go to the Cancer Center for an appointment once, but they sat in the lobby. Grace did come to Mayo when I had my surgery which we had not planned on, but she just really needed to be there. They also went to a plastic surgery appointment with Doug and I once as we were traveling through Rochester. Even though they did not really attend any appointments, they were very aware of what was happening and we were pretty honest with them about my prognosis and what I could and could not do during treatment.

JUST KEEPIN' ON KEEPIN' ON

JOURNAL ENTRY BY HEIDI EDWARDS
SEPTEMBER 18, 2017

Last week was decent, but Avery got a bad cold that I ended up sharing with her. It is resolving itself, and I was still able to get treatment today. :)

Grace did indeed have a fractured little toe, so she is not able to run at least through this week, maybe longer. (I will take her for another x-ray on Friday.) She can still ride an exercise bike and go to the weight room, though, and is attending practices. She took pictures for the school newspaper at Friday's football game and cheered on her cross country team at Saturday's meet.

Lauren and Ave are adjusting to middle school, and had their second cross country meet on Thursday. It was a little rougher than the first meet. It was really hot, in the mid 80's, and Ave was still struggling with the cold. (Lauren thought she had a little one as well.) They were nervous, but Grace told them there were only two rules for the race.

1. Finish the race.
2. Don't cry.

They mostly followed the rules, and they finished the race. There was a little crying. Doug is hanging tough. He worked hard all week, and by the time Friday rolled around, he WAS DONE.

The first Taxol treatment went smoothly with no negative drug reactions and nausea was not a problem. I was tired, but I also had a cold.

Today was the second treatment. My friend, RaeAnn, went with me. As of today, I am halfway through treatment with chemotherapy. I had eight weeks of A/C treatment and I just finished two weeks of Taxol. That is twenty weeks total, and I am done with TEN!!

I got a nurse to take a pic of us holding a sign that said:

TAXOL—#2 of 12 Treatments—9/18/17—with RaeAnn

The nurse seemed kind of confused, and I explained that I was halfway through with chemo. She looked at my sign, and said, "Two of twelve is not halfway."

I tried to explain to her, but she still didn't seem to understand.

It's OK, RaeAnn and I understood, and I think a person has to CELEBRATE EVERY MILESTONE in a cancer journey.

WHAT TO DO WHEN YOU ARE DONE, BUT NOT DONE—LEAN ON YOUR FAITH, YOUR FAMILY, AND YOUR FRIENDS

JOURNAL ENTRY BY HEIDI EDWARDS
SEPTEMBER 25, 2017

It's 4:45 a.m. on Treatment Day #3 of Taxol. I woke up about an hour ago, and stayed in bed for half an hour before I decided to just get up already. I started a load of laundry and tried to empty the dishwasher, but when I opened it the detergent pack was sticking to the side of the inside door. I started it again on the "Quick Cycle".

Yesterday afternoon I decided I was sick of this whole cancer deal. Plus, I have been fasting for 24 hours before each treatment, and I was hangry (hungry and angry). While I was serving up dinner with sort of a smile, Lauren was complaining that it "just didn't look too tasty" to her. I will admit it was the same thing she had for lunch, but COME ON!

"Lauren," I said, "you are just so lucky that you are having a nice, hot tasty dinner. I cannot EVEN LISTEN to any complaints. EAT IT."

"I'm not really hungry now either," Avery shared.

"If you don't want to eat now, you are NOT eating junk and snacking later," I replied.

"Honey," Doug said to me, "you seem a little crabby, maybe you should eat."

"Geez, Dad, you are such a man," Grace chimed in.

"I'm fine, just fine," I said. And I was fine, just DONE with treatment, but NOT done. After Doug cleaned up the dinner dishes, we went for a walk (we have a neighborhood loop) and when I returned to the house, I was in a much better place.

Really, I am OK. I am OK because I have my FAITH, my FAMILY, and my FRIENDS with me. That doesn't mean I don't wish I could just be done with all this cancer crap, but I AM OK. I have my.................

Faith—

I will keep my eyes on the Lord. With Him at my right hand, I will not be shaken. Psalm 16:8

Those who trust in the Lord will find new strength. Isaiah 40:31

I know the plans I have for you, says the Lord, plans to prosper and not to harm you, plans to give you hope and a future. Jeremiah 29:11

At the end of the day, I KNOW God has me in his Hands. I KNOW that He will give me strength for this journey.

Ok, now I am tired again, so I am going to lay on the sofa with the Wonder Woman blanket some of my prayer warriors gave me. And—Up again...........

The girls are all off to school. Praise the Lord for school. I mean, truly, PRAISE THE LORD and God bless all the men and women who dedicate their lives to this noble calling.

Ok, back to the main point of this post. In addition to my faith, I could not have gotten to this point in this journey (in the relatively strong physical and emotional place I am) without ....

Family—

Thank you to my Mom and Dad for being rocks for us. They have come up whenever we needed them and mowed the lawn, cooked, cleaned, done DIY projects with the girls, made applesauce, shopped, gone to horse lessons, gone thrifting, gone shopping, and on and on. We are giving them a little break now because we are doing OK. They are home in Iowa catching up on their own lives. We will need them again, and I know they will come.

My dear sweet Doug has walked right alongside me during this time, and has been my biggest advocate and cheerleader. He has dragged me off the sofa and up Rib Mountain time after time. He has read books and articles on how to beat this and called about clinical trials for me. He has ordered supplements for me and encouraged me to drastically change my diet. He has prayed over me almost every night. He has spent as much time as he can with me because we both feel better when we are together.

My sweet girls are in this with me, too. Last night, in bed, Avery said, "Mom, did you know October is Breast Cancer Awareness month? Isn't that cool?" Lauren and Grace wanted bracelets like mine that say "Stand up to Cancer". G found a pink ribbon pin at a thrift shop to wear on her black Under Armour hat.

Friends—

I HAVE BEEN BLESSED BEYOND MEASURE BY ALL THE FRIENDS IN MY LIFE. Thank you to all of you for the cards, the meals, the gifts, the flowers, the blankets, the gift cards, the rides to treatments and sitting with me during treatment. Thank you to those of you who have had the girls over for playdates and taken them to horse lessons, and to and from practice when needed. Thank you to the folks who participated in the Susan G. Komen with us. Thank you for the texts and the calls and the visits. Thank you to those of you who have left encouraging messages on the CaringBridge site. Thanks to my college friends for the t-shirts. All these acts of love have CHANGED the course of this journey for me and for my family. They are undoubtedly the greatest gifts I HAVE EVER RECEIVED.

OK, now I am going to unload that dishwasher, fold the clothes in the dryer, and get ready for treatment today. PAUSE——PAUSE—-PAUSE

Back from treatment and all went well.

Love you all—Heidi

Reflection

The Five F's That Got Me Through: Faith, Family, Friends, Fitness, and Food

Faith is a belief that he who began this good work in me will bring it to completion.

Faith is being sure of what you hope for, and certain of what you cannot see.

Faith is believing that all things work for good for those who love the Lord.

Choose faith over fear.

OK, this is a tough pill to swallow, but faith does not always mean physical healing. I have been so blessed that up until this point (today being the end of 2021) that I have experienced physical healing. But what if I had not? Where would my faith be? Would I still be able to share these verses? I hope and I pray that my answer would be YES. And the truth is that none of us ever know if tomorrow we or someone we love will be in a life-threatening situation.

Family and Friends

Family and friends are the hands and feet of Jesus. Family and friends provide the support that people need to survive during times of all difficulty, not just during times of health crises. It was family and friends who sustained me, physically, emotionally, and spiritually. Physically, I was so blessed with meals and rides (to chemo for me and to school/other events for the girls). I also had a few friends who made the trek to Mayo with me. I was blessed with gift cards and blankets and other gifts too numerous to mention. I had Catholic friends who gifted me with necklaces of the patron saints of healing. My dentist friend, Denise, gave me the appropriate mouthwash and sugar free candy to suck on. My personal trainer friend, Sarah, devised a work out for me during chemo. Another friend, Andrea, blessed me with hats.

Emotionally, I was blessed with calls and texts, letters and hugs. I had a friend, Amy, who organized the Hooters for Heidi team for Susan G. Komen. My college friends also designed a t-shirt. The rest of the suite-mates purchased one and sent me pics of themselves wearing them. As I write this, I am aware of the fact that not everyone has a wide network of social support. What do you do if this is your situation?

Tap into whatever you've got, baby. Family, work friends, church friends, neighbors—accept help from whoever offers help. Sometimes other survivors step forward and offer to help. Most cancer centers have a social worker that might help "fill in the gaps". You need help. You can't do it alone. People are good. People show up for each other.

Side Note: I also know that not everyone is coming from a place of financial security. I am pretty darn lucky that I did not have to add financial worry to the long list of things people worry about during health crises. Financial insecurity is not my situation right now, but I get it. As I was writing this reflection, I came across a few organizations that seem reputable. My guess is that the social worker at the spot where the patient is receiving care would be the best spot to inquire about financial assistance.

CancerCare Co-Payment Assistance Foundation

According to the website, "We help people with cancer overcome financial access and treatment barriers by assisting them with co-payments for their prescribed treatments. We offer easy-to-access, same-day approval over the phone and online."

Patient Access Network Foundation (PANF) Toll-free number: 1-866-316-7263

Pan Foundation

Website: www.panfoundation.org

Helps under-insured patients with certain cancer diagnoses cover out-of-pocket costs related to cancer care.

Leukemia and Lymphoma Society

If you are dealing with leukemia or lymphoma, this is another reputable organization.

Leukemia & Lymphoma Society at 1-800-955-4572 or look on www. lls.org.

I did not take advantage of this cleaning service, but I know women and men who have accessed this organization.

Cleaning for a Reason

877-337-3348

I know that I have not even scratched the surface of organizations that can assist cancer patients. The point is that assistance is available and that getting through a cancer diagnosis and treatment is so much easier with the help of family and friends. You have to ask, though, because people don't necessarily know if you are in need. Your local treatment center is a great place to start.

Fitness

Ok, this is just my two cents worth on fitness during cancer. Moving my body and making my body work physically during treatment was HUGE. I actually improved my physical fitness during treatment and post-surgery. I really didn't do anything fancy. I just walked. That's it. I walked. I walked around my neighborhood. I walked in Wal-Mart. I used my grandma's trick of parking farther away from the building I was entering and got a few extra steps that way. I walked at the quarry and at Rib Mountain State Park. I walked at Mayo while I was in-between appointments. I did work a bit with my friend, Sarah, who is a personal trainer, but you don't need a personal trainer. Almost everyone has a smart phone these days and you can find some easy strength training exercises to do at home, maybe even with soup cans for light weights. Our YMCA also offers a program called Livestrong for cancer survivors that I believe is free of charge. Exercising during cancer treatment and after cancer treatment is powerful physical medicine and powerful emotional medicine. Exercise gives you autonomy over your body and reminds you that just because you have cancer in one area of your body, the rest of your body IS STILL HEALTHY. Also, as I mentioned previously, exercise can protect your body against the damaging effects of chemo and release powerful mood enhancing chemicals. When you exercise, your body releases chemicals called endorphins. Doug tells me the endorphins communicate with your brain receptors and lower your pain perception. Endorphins also improve mood. So, there you have it folks, inasmuch as humanly possible, move!

Food

Ok, again, this is just my two cents worth on food and nutrition during chemo as I AM NOT a nutritionist or a doctor. When people are initially diagnosed with cancer, I think many people, myself included, ask themselves if "their diet contributed to their cancer diagnosis". Hmmmmm….. That is probably like going down a rabbit hole. I had a pretty normal BMI until my mid-twenties at which point I struggled mightily with anxiety. I started on some SSRIs (selective serotonin reuptake inhibitors) and gained a fair bit of weight. In retrospect, the SSRIs did contribute to my weight gain, but so did a steady diet of restaurant food and other poor food choices. I battled my weight on and off for about 20 years (mostly on), until, oddly enough, I managed to lose 20 pounds right before I was diagnosed. I still wonder if the weight loss allowed me to find the lump or if the weight loss caused a metabolic shift that contributed to the cancer developing. (There is absolutely nothing scientific about my theory, but when you develop cancer, you have all these crazy theories about what might have caused it.)

Anyway, moving away from these unanswerable questions……. The real point I am trying to make is that I was still 25 pounds overweight at the time of diagnosis. Immediately upon being diagnosed, I analyzed every bite I put into my body and felt like anything "unhealthy" was causing the cancer cells to grow exponentially. Soda, chips, candy, baked goods, deli meat, processed carbs, cheese, and diet soda all lost their appeal and almost made me gag. The first several weeks post-diagnosis I lost weight quickly, and then it leveled out. I ate lots of fruits and vegetables and we started buying organic as much as possible. We were already buying organic milk, and we continued. Of course, the way I was eating is the way I should have been eating even prior to a cancer diagnosis.

The American Cancer Society's website cancer.org is a treasure trove of information and I appreciated their no-nonsense advice for navigating nutrition during treatment. I am sharing from the article "Eating Well During Treatment". I am quoting directly:

Try to eat well. A healthy diet helps your body function at its best. This is even more important if you have cancer. You'll go into treatment with reserves to help keep up your strength, your energy level, and your defenses against infection. A healthy diet can also prevent body tissue from breaking down and build new tissues. People who eat well are better able to cope with side effects of treatment. And you may even be able to handle higher doses of certain drugs. In fact, some cancer treatments work better in people who are well-nourished and are getting enough calories and protein. Try these tips:

Don't be afraid to try new foods. Some things you never have liked before might taste good during treatment.

Choose different plant-based foods. Try eating beans and peas instead of meat at a few meals each week.

- Try to eat more fruits and vegetables every day, including citrus fruits and dark-green and deep-yellow vegetables. Colorful vegetables and fruits and plant-based foods have many natural health-promoting substances.
- Try to stay at a healthy weight, and stay physically active. Small weight changes during treatment are normal.
- Limit the amount of salt-cured, smoked, and pickled foods you eat.
- Limit or avoid red or processed meats

If you can't do any of the above during this time, don't worry about it. Help is available if or when you need it. Tell your cancer care team about any problems you have. Sometimes diet changes are needed to get the extra fluids, protein, and calories you need.

A follow-up article, "Tips for Healthy Eating After Cancer Treatment", also at cancer.org from the American Cancer Society discusses diet once your treatment is over. Again, I am quoting directly from the article:

Check with your cancer care team to see if you have any food or diet restrictions.

Ask your dietitian to help you create a nutritious, balanced eating plan.

Try to eat a variety of colorful fruits and vegetables each day; include citrus fruits and dark-green and deep-yellow vegetables.

Eat plenty of high-fiber foods, like whole-grain breads and cereals.

Try to buy a different fruit, vegetable, low-fat food, or whole-grain product each time you shop for groceries.

Avoid or limit your intake of red meat (beef, pork, or lamb) and processed meats such as salt-cured, smoked, and pickled foods (including bacon, sausage, and deli meats).

Choose low-fat milk and dairy products.

It is best not to drink alcohol. If you drink, limit the amount to no more than 1 drink per day for women, and 2 for men. Alcohol is a known cancer-causing agent.

My beloved oncologist, Dr. Anand, told me that I did not need to do anything radical during or post-treatment. He recommended a Mediterranean diet. I understand that to be a diet rich in veggies, fruits, legumes, nuts, whole grains, fish, and unsaturated fats. Red meat and dairy is consumed minimally. Sugar and processed meats are avoided. He also told me that the past was the past and worrying about my past consumption of "unhealthy" foods wasn't going to help me move forward and deal with my present reality. And so, because I did believe cleaning up my diet would help my body "fight" the cancer AND because it gave me a sense of control, I did make a conscious effort to follow the guidelines mentioned above. In the process, I did lose some weight and I do believe that I tolerated treatment better. Most importantly, I felt like I was doing what I COULD to GET BETTER and fight the cancer.

Just a disclaimer here: There were times, especially the day right after chemo, when I could only eat carbs. I was able to tolerate baked potatoes with a little butter. So, you tolerate what you can, but, when and if you can, use food as medicine and choose foods that strengthen and support your health.

SLOW AND STEADY, BUT REALLY FAST, TOO

Journal Entry by Heidi Edwards
October 2, 2017

From a treatment perspective, things are just slow and steady. I had my fourth Taxol treatment this morning, and my great friend/neighbor, Jennifer, drove me and kept me company. The infusion room was BUSY. There were lots of patients receiving treatment and the nurses were just trying to keep up with it all. God bless them! My friend Amy R. (who works as a nurse at the hospital right next door to the Cancer Center) bopped over during her break and brought me a chemo crown. The crown she presented me with has nine little heads of my oncologist. After each treatment, I can take off a head. I wish I could move this part of my life a little more quickly, but no go. Kudos to these friends for keeping me company and making me laugh.

Even though treatment isn't going fast enough, a lot of life is moving at breakneck speed. Saturday morning the twins and I met a good friend at a new coffee shop. G had homecoming this weekend (shortened to hoco in teenage vernacular). We had 13 girls over to get ready and then another mom and I took them to dinner before the dance. (When they all left, the upstairs smelled like a mix of hairspray, perfume, and sweat.) Doug opened all the windows to air out the second story. I honestly think Lauren and Avery and their two buddies had as much fun watching the girls get ready as the girls had getting ready.

On Sunday, we went to church and a birthday party for the children of some good friends. It was a "Trucks and Tiaras" party for a four and six-year-old. It was a great party with tiaras for the girls, a bounce house, bubbles, presents and TWO cakes. Doug took Lauren to Pier One last night because, in her words "the fall sale is ending today, and I still need a decorative pillow to complete my room". (She has been redecorating her room since June.) We tried to explain to her that there is ALWAYS A SALE, but she didn't believe us.

OCTOBER MAGIC

JOURNAL ENTRY BY HEIDI EDWARDS
OCTOBER 9, 2017

I don't know why, but September is not my favorite month. I often reference the song, "Wake Me Up When September Ends" when I am in the midst of September.

Maybe it is because summer is over, and it takes all of us (Doug, me, and the kids) a while to accept that fact and realize that the school year is going to be a lot of hard work and early mornings. We have to mourn that fact for a while before just dealing with it, and GETTING TO WORK. September also means new routines, swapping out the summer clothes for winter clothes, and closing up the cabin. This year, when September started, I also still had a lot of chemo left.

Interestingly, I read on-line that the song referenced above was written by Green Day lead singer Billie Joe Armstrong about his dad, who died of cancer on September 1, 1982. After the funeral, he locked himself in his room, and said, "Wake me up when September ends."

SEPTEMBER IS OVER, AND NOW IS IT OCTOBER, THOUGH. I love October. The air is crisp, the leaves are falling, and the sky just seems so blue. I love how the sun warms my body through jeans and a jacket. We have had a great October so far.

Last Thursday, I got to speak (for a few minutes) at a Volley for the Cure event at the high school where Grace goes. The two high schools in town, West and East competed in the name of raising money for Breast Cancer Awareness. (It is perfect timing as October is Breast Cancer Awareness month.) Obviously, this is planned and not just random timing.

Also last Thursday, Lauren and Avery had a cross country meet. G was able to run on Saturday in the rain. It was her first race post broken toe. I love, love, love watching cross country meets and cheering for all the runners, fast or slow or somewhere in the middle. On Saturday evening, the girls harvested all the pumpkins from our little garden (about 30), washed them, and arranged them by our front door.

On Sunday, we went to an apple orchard. We did a corn maze, picked some apples, fed the goats, and waited in a ridiculously long line for cinnamon ice cream and a pumpkin donut. Also, Lauren and I (and a friend) rode the "cow train".

Today my friend, AR, (just her initials here) took me to treatment. She jazzed up the event by presenting me with a lot of Breast Cancer Awareness items from the Dollar Store. That woman is AWESOME and I was looking FINE during my Taxol.

I am done with Treatment #5. Only 7 more to go!

Reflection

One interesting and extremely meaningful thing that happened during treatment was the people who reached out to me that I hadn't necessarily had a close connection to before my diagnosis. AR was one of these people. She just showed up. She had some unique connections to my situation. For one, she is a nurse, so she gets the medical piece of all of it. I think she even did some work in oncology at one time. Secondly, she lost her own mom to breast cancer. What is so amazing to me was how AR just showed up. I know if I told her that she would brush it off, but it is true. She has a wicked sense of humor, too, and a sense of humor helps most situations. I also made some connections to some other folks uniquely because of breast cancer that I will discuss in another post.

CROSS COUNTRY AND CANCER

Journal Entry by Heidi Edwards
October 16, 2017

Last week we had a lot of cross country ACTION at our house.

My mom and dad came up just in time to watch Lauren and Avery run their conference meet on Tuesday after school and stayed until Saturday to watch G run her conference meet. They also helped us A LOT during their visit. Once they arrived from Iowa on Tuesday, we loaded up in my van and headed over to the middle school on the east side of town (we're west-siders) for the meet. When we got there, we found the girls and they seemed, borrowing from G's vernacular, pretty chill. They were so engaged in snapping photos with their friends (for Instagram posts) that they barely had time to come over and say hi to Doug, me, or Papa and Grammy. I would not describe their demeanor as nervous. In fact, I was worried they might not make it over to the starting line. But, they did. And, they ran well. Their improvement (both mentally and physically) since the first race was striking. Ave finished 91 out of 155 runners and Lauren 102 out of 155. It was a happy day for them and for us. We were so happy because there was no CRYING AT ALL and because they did something THEY DIDN'T THINK THEY COULD DO AT THE BEGINNING OF THE YEAR. They deserve to be called athletes now.

G bounced back from her broken toe! She ran last week in Merrill and this week she ran JV at the Conference Meet. She finished 14 out of 104 runners and watching her run the last 800 meters was just beautiful and thrilling. I was so proud of her for sticking with the season and being patient and doing what she could do even when she couldn't run.

I ran cross country in high school, too. Middle school cross country didn't exist in my district at that time. Looking back, it was one of the most rewarding things I did in high school. This wasn't because I was particularly talented. In fact, my freshmen year, I actually finished DEAD LAST in one race. I got better though, and by the time I was a senior, I could finish the two-mile race (now girls run a 5K in high school) in under 14 minutes.

I think a cross country race has a lot of similarities to a cancer journey. At the beginning of both experiences, a person's emotions are very heightened. There is so much apprehension. What will the outcome ultimately be? Will I have the physical strength for the journey? Will I have the mental strength for the journey?

In cross country, you hope for an outcome based on achieving a certain time or place position. With cancer, you hope for a "cure" or to live a high quality of life as long as possible.

In cross country, you hope that you will have the physical strength to achieve your outcome. You hope that you will be able to run with the least amount of pain possible and that you have strength at the end to "finish strong". With cancer (during chemo), you pray for energy and for "good blood counts" and (in my case) that you avoid neuropathy and mouth sores. You also pray that you can complete treatment with the least amount of pain possible and that you have the physical strength to "finish strong".

In cross country, you hope for the emotional strength to keep going even when you are done. With cancer, you hope for the emotional strength to keep going even when you are done.

Cross country and cancer are also the same in that in both "races" there are people cheering you on, there is an endpoint, and you are a different person after each race.

One of the best parts of cross country is the support the runners receive from the spectators. All the runners get encouragement, not just the fastest competitors. In fact, sometimes the last runners get the most support. In cancer, the support that I have received has literally humbled me beyond measure. I have had so many folks "cheering me on".

In cross country, there is an end—the finish line. At the conference meet, runners crossed that line in different ways. Some finished with strength left. Some gave it everything they had, but were still able to walk with a bit of support. At the conference meet, there was a runner (from West) who literally crawled across the finish line. (God bless that girl!) I think cancer is like that, too. There will be an endpoint. I am hopeful that the end for me will be a successful treatment and a long life. I know that for some the endpoint is just more time, and for some the endpoint is passage to another life. As a believer, I believe that once I pass from this life, I will be with Jesus.

Finally, in both races, the participants are different after the race. In cross country, most runners are glad they had the experience, happy to be finished, and proud of what they have accomplished. Even though they might not have wanted to run the race, they are DIFFERENT afterwards—in a GOOD WAY. I do not have the post-cancer perspective yet, but I hope I will be different afterwards—in a GOOD WAY. I know that for many patients, they may not be able to find good from it, particularly depending on the outcome. That said, no matter what the outcome is for me, I am working hard to find blessings from this.

I know that all sports are unique and very meaningful, but you can probably tell that I am a wee bit partial to this sport. I believe that it will help my daughters, and all the participants to LEARN THAT THEY ARE STRONGER THAN THEY THINK THEY ARE. From this experience, they will be a little bit more prepared to take on life's challenges. Also—a big shout out to WEST—GOOD LUCK AT SECTIONALS ON FRIDAY!!

On a side note, I am halfway through my twelve-week regimen of Taxol. My good friend and former neighbor, Mary, sat with me during treatment today. I am hanging tough, and running strong.

And let us run with perseverance the race marked out for us, fixing our eyes on Jesus, the pioneer and perfecter of our faith. Hebrews 12:1-2

Reflection

OK, I am still biased and I think cross country is the BEST SPORT EVER. Grace ran all four years of high school, and Lauren and Avery ran with her as ninth graders this year. Lauren is running right now, and Avery is taking a year off to focus on finishing up the Youth Horse Development Program with the American Quarter Horse Association.

BRACELETS, BLANKETS, HILLS, AND HORSES— SOURCES OF STRENGTH

JOURNAL ENTRY BY HEIDI EDWARDS
OCTOBER 23, 2017

Since I was diagnosed in July, I have been gifted with a number of unique, beautiful BRACELETS—all of which I wear EVERY SINGLE DAY—even to bed. I take one of them off to shower, but I let the rest of them get wet. I cherish them and the people who gave them to me because they make me feel loved. Three are Alex and Ani bracelets and they jingle a little bit on my wrist and dance when I move. Another is a wooden beaded bracelet. (I got two like this, and gave one to Grace.) There is another that simply says strength. My two aunts gave me a beautiful one with beads and a little heart box with a prayer inside. I did take the prayer out because I don't want it to get wet. There is another that is made of three leather strips. One strip says FAITH. Another says BE THE LIGHT. SHINE. The third says BELIEVE IN MIRACLES. This leather bracelet is the one I take off to shower. (I hope I am not missing any. If I am, forgive me.)

I have also been gifted with BLANKETS. My mom was the first to give me a blanket, a small, soft pink blanket that probably only weighs ounces and feels like a feather when it is covering me. She gave it to me when I went to Mayo. Then two blankets in a box from Amazon came. One of them is also very light and the softness of it reminds me of a very gentle breeze when I use it. Then another "mom" (someone who mothered me) from my childhood sent a plaid purple, pink, and black blanket that she made. Some ladies from church/school moms gave me a Wonder Woman blanket that I covered up in the recliner with after the Adriamycin/Cytoxan treatment this summer. We also got a cozy, colorful Vera Bradley throw from a friend of Grace's. Today, a dear woman, Ms. Stacy, gave me a quilt she made with different colors of gray and pink and

I was OVERWHELMED. I have literally been covered in love and prayers. Those of you who know me well know that I am a "tosser" and I don't keep things that I don't need anymore, but I am telling you that I will keep these blankets FOREVER. Someday, my forty-year-old daughters will be at my house, looking at these blankets, and say, "C'mon, Mom, get rid of them. We will get you some new ones." And, I will refuse, because they will represent a time in my life when I was held.

These have been tangible sources of strength. A non-tangible source of strength for me has been walking every day that I can. My favorite place to walk is Rib Mountain. (It is really like a big HILL, but Marathon County natives call it a mountain.) The mountain is almost four miles long and peaks at 1,942 above sea level. When I walk, I don't walk quite up to the top; I walk up to the Ranger Station, and then turn around which is a little over three miles in total. It is a great cardio workout, and I have never once regretted walking. We all (the whole family) went last night right at dusk, and it was nearly dark by the time we got back to the car. The walking path was almost completely covered with red, orange, and yellow leaves. We were content to walk and talk and Doug, Lauren, and Ave took turns walking Louise. We stopped at the top and from the north side of the mountain we could see most of Wausau. I feel stronger and calmer each time I walk here.

Moving on to other sources of strength, horses.........

I should be honest, horses aren't actually a source of strength for me, but they are for Avery. Horses were a big part of the weekend for Doug and Ave; I wanted to just have a little fun and mention how her horse weekend played out. She was able to participate in a Pleasure Fun Show on Saturday. She and Doug were at the barn (where she takes lessons) to load up Bailey (the horse she used) by 6:30 a.m. They weren't back home until 6:30 that night. None of us knew what to expect, but Avery, in the words of her riding instructor "did so great". She came home with some ribbons and a desire to "do more shows"! Doug came home saying "horse people are pretty good people". All the other people from the barn showed him love and offered him a chair, lunch, snacks and pretty good conversation. He also learned what a mare, gelding, and stallion are. I think he was a pretty darn good horse dad this weekend!

On another side note, I had my seventh of twelve TAXOL treatments today. My friend, Stacy (the blanket Stacy), went with me and we had such a good chat I was actually a little sorry the time went by so quickly. My blood counts were still OK, and I am praying that they stay high enough that I can get all treatments with no delays.

Signing off with love—Heidi

Reflection

I still have all of those bracelets. I don't wear them anymore because I don't need them anymore. They are in a bag, and the bag is in the top drawer of a little side table in my bedroom closet. Every once in a while, I open the drawer and pick up the bag. I take out each bracelet one by one and hold each bracelet in the palm of my hand. Even though none of them weigh much, they feel solid in my hands, and I still gather strength from them.

We have the blankets as well and they are used on a daily basis, and they are readily accessible in a built-in cupboard in our living room. I wash them about once a month because we use them when we are studying, watching TV, napping, or just relaxing. We will keep them until they fall apart. I know who gave me each blanket.

We don't walk the hill as much anymore, but we still walk a lot. We walk more in our neighborhood or my new personal favorite spot, the dog park. The girls don't walk with us much anymore, and I am a little sad about that. I can sometimes talk one of them into a walk with me, but usually it is just Doug and Louise.

Horses, well, the horse situation has exploded. Avery (really Doug and I) bought Rusty in December of 2019. In the summer of 2020, Avery applied for a position in the Youth Horse Development Program through the American Quarter Horse Association. Applicants who are accepted receive a weanling (from adult members) and agree to participate in a nine-month program. At the completion of the program, the applicant gets to keep the horse. Avery was accepted, and at the end of October, Doug, Avery, Lauren and Avery's friend, E, traveled to South Dakota to pick up Lux. Avery is (basically) responsible for supporting Lux financially. Horses continue to be a huge source of strength and community for her. She recently sold Rusty, and purchased a new quarter horse named Cutie Pie that has been renamed Lola. Doug and I spend a lot of time at the barn, sitting with her, talking to the other barn folks, and occasionally helping out with chores.

NYC

Journal Entry by Heidi Edwards
October 30, 2017

One of the things I love most in this life is travel. I am fascinated by leaving what I know and going to what I don't know. I love planning for trips, going on trips, and remembering and recording trips. As a child, I made scrapbooks of the places I had been. I pasted brochures, receipts, and memorabilia next to my own written recollections of trips in paper scrapbooks my Mom bought for me. I am sure my creations weren't that interesting to anyone but me, but I didn't care because they were a documentation of my experiences. I didn't make them for anyone except myself.

Last March, before I could have even imagined what my life would be like in October, we planned a trip to New York City over our short Fall Break. When I was diagnosed in early July, we weren't sure what to do about the trip, so we did nothing. We decided to take a "wait and see" approach. We had gotten the airplane tickets with credit card points, and at most, we would only have to pay for one night at the hotel. (We could cancel the other nights.)

With cancer, I have been afraid to plan too far ahead or make commitments. It feels like things are too uncertain. When I make plans with family or friends, I always add an "if" statement. "I would love to come if......" What's the if? If I feel well enough, if I am not sick, if you are not sick, if I am not exhausted by that time of day .... Cancer has taken some of the certainty out of my life. It is a little foolish, really, because none of us really has certainty. We don't know what our life will look like in a few months.

So, even last weekend, I still wasn't 100% sure if the trip would be a go, but we did pack our bags and I bought tickets to see the Statue of Liberty and Ellis Island and the 9/11 Museum. That was all I bought, though, because I just didn't want to waste money if we couldn't go. BUT, last Tuesday, we set off for Minneapolis and I found a hotel (on the car trip) for us to stay in before our flight the next morning. We checked in—Doug and I slept in one bed, Grace and Ave in another, and Lauren on the new Aerobed. By nine the next morning, we were on the plane. I had a blue mask on, and Doug and I were still a little bit unsure about whether or not traveling to NYC was a good idea.

As it turned out, it WAS A GOOD IDEA. There were whole hours that went by without a thought of cancer passing through my head. Doug said the same was true for him. We saw the Statue of Liberty and Ellis Island. We saw the 9/11 Museum and the Empire State Building. We saw a little girl get bit by a squirrel she was hand-feeding peanuts to. (We called that one before it happened. I think her French parents thought the park was like a petting zoo. We told them not to feed the squirrel, but they didn't listen.) We saw the sister-in-law and niece of some of our best friends in Wausau. They took the train from Long Island to meet us for BBQ. During the trip, we walked A LOT, and I was tired, but we were in our room early all but one of the nights. In addition to all the things mentioned above, we saw Central Park and I sat in the sun and just let the warmth soak into me. We saw lots of interesting people and ate some great food. I saw that life will (very, very likely) be normal again and that I don't need to be afraid to keep moving forward and making plans.

The night before we left, we saw the musical *Hamilton*. If you haven't seen it, the musical is basically about the private and personal life of one of the Founding Fathers, Alexander Hamilton. I was entranced the whole time, but the second act, and particularly the ending, just brought me to tears. Throughout the whole musical, there is a theme of legacy and how the life stories of people are remembered. At the end, when Hamilton is killed in a duel, that theme is expressed in the song *Who Lives? Who Dies? Who Tells Your Story?* written by Lin-Manuel Miranda. (Lyrics cannot be cited due to copyright, but look them up, they are AMAZING.)

As I listened to the song hot, heavy tears ran down my face, smudging my mascara, and threatening to turn into all out sobbing. The song evoked the reality that we are all mortal, and made me wonder about my own story and whether I have done enough, and whether I would live to be old.

I can honestly say that I think I will be fine and that I will not die from breast cancer, but you CANNOT go through this experience without going to that place in your mind. You just CANNOT. You cannot go through this experience wondering if you have done enough and what you still need to do.

Maybe the trick is not staying in that place for too long. Maybe the trick is moving forward and making plans. Maybe the trick is holding your breath and hoping.

On a happy note.....I had the 8th of 12 TAXOL treatments today. I only have 4 weeks of treatment left. Another Amy went with me. She is a dear soul who is upbeat and funny and joyful, and her presence was a gift. For all you prayer warriors out there, keep praying that I can on course and finish the treatments on time. Oh—and for no neuropathy! (Blood counts look fine right now.)

With love and thanks-Heidi

Reflection

Well, I got to see *Hamilton* again with my Mom and Dad in Des Moines, Iowa, the summer after treatment and it was just as good the second time around. My dad can't hear very well, so he couldn't pick up on the humor and the nuances and the sheer creative genius in Hamilton. That made me a little sad because he is a huge history buff.

I loved the songs as much the second time, especially the lyrics *"Who Lives, Who Dies, Who Tells Your Story"*. Again, they are like poetry, and they always bring me to tears.

As I wrote in the original CaringBridge post, the first time I saw *Hamilton,* I left the theatre dumbstruck. After the production in NYC, Grace called Hamilton "life changing" and I agree with her. It was life-changing for me the first time I heard it, especially because I was still in active treatment for cancer.

One very surreal thing about cancer is that it gives you a chance (is chance the right word) to ponder the question asked in the *Hamilton* song mentioned above.

Once you leave the earth, who remembers you? Have you done what you needed to do?

I thought about that a lot. Mostly, I worried about my girls and if they would remember my name. I wondered if I had taught them enough? Had I done enough for them? What if I missed their graduations? What if I missed their weddings? What if I never saw them as mothers? When I sat in that theatre chair, in the span of time it took for the artists to sing the song, all of these thoughts passed through my mind.

I wondered if and when Doug would get married again if I died. He said he wouldn't, but honestly, it seems like most men do. I guess a lot of women do too, because someone is marrying the widowers. I thought about another woman in my house and tried to imagine who I would pick for Doug. I always think I wouldn't get remarried if Doug died; I would be OK as a single lady. My maternal grandmother lost her husband in her thirties and never got remarried. My mother-in-law lost her husband before she was fifty, and 18 years later, she is still single. I guess you just never know though what you would really do if you were in that situation. Would you find love again? Maybe......maybe not.......

Of course, at the time, I knew I hadn't done enough for them, because parents never really feel like they have done enough, do they?

And if you lose a parent to cancer so early, what does it do to kids? I was sad to die for myself, but I was more sad for my kids because no one loves a kid (except for their dad) like their mom does. I know that kids thrive and move forward and they are OK. My own mom was one of those kids. But still..........

HOW BEAUTIFUL THE HANDS THAT SERVE

JOURNAL ENTRY BY HEIDI EDWARDS
NOVEMBER 6, 2017

How beautiful the hands that (have served)............

1. The turkey/beef meatloaf that everyone in the family described as "comfort food"

2. The Zuppa Tuscana (Tuscan Soup) from D that we ate outside on a warm September night and the Chicken Noodle soup that we ate on a cold October night with rolls from The Mint (a local restaurant)

3. The Morning Glory Bread chock full of goodness and tastiness and the generous serving of soup that came with it (so good Grace licked the bowl)

4. The "make your own pizza" ingredients, including a gluten free crust

5. The tender Mexican pot roast with just the right amount of spice for us Midwesterners (with all the fixings) and the beautiful already sliced meatloaf with onions, potatoes, carrots

6. The BBQ ribs and mashed potatoes that fed us almost three meals

7. The Mexican lasagna and chicken lasagna and "Mom's recipe" lasagna and the amazing HUGE lasagna

8. The spaghetti and meatballs delivered by a mom and her four-year-old

9. The fruit salads (G's favorite) and lettuce salads with yummy croutons and awesome dressings

10. The fresh fish caught by two of the best fishermen I know (father and son combo) and the salmon and halibut from Alaska

11. The hot, cheesy pizza from a favorite local spot close to our house
12. The tender pork tenderloin worthy of being called gourmet with beautiful sides to compliment the meal
13. The pork carnitas and chicken tacos with Qdoba style additions (veggies, cheese, sour cream and guacamole)
14. The fresh salads, one with feta and quinoa and Kalamata olives
15. The hot beef sandwiches with cheese, peppers, onions and mushrooms
16. The pulled pork (twice) once with baked beans and coleslaw, once with beans and cheesy potatoes AND the grilled chicken and grilled potatoes
17. The quiche and the keto chicken, keto bagels and fresh cucumbers
18. The hot ham and cheese sandwiches enjoyed on Memorial Day and the beef enchiladas enjoyed after Lauren and Ave's parent/teacher conferences
19. The containers of feta and Kalamata olives from Elisabeth who now lives in Milwaukee and the chicken dumpling casserole with a fun sweet salad to go along with
20. The brownies, cookies, pies, bars, zucchini bread, pumpkin bread, banana bread, and other treats

There were so many other wonderful meals that showed up on our kitchen table and "filled us up" both physically and spiritually.

Changing gears........................

From the moment a woman becomes a mother, she starts nurturing her child. She rocks her child, she changes her child, she holds her child, AND......she feeds her child. Initially, she either breast feeds, bottle feeds or a combo of both. Eventually, she moves on to baby food, and then, she begins to prepare meal after meal after meal. Maybe her family grows to have more children, maybe not, but one thing stays certain. Her children and husband (or maybe not if she is a single mom) keep eating and that means shopping, prepping, cooking, and cleaning up. Some partners cook, but that has never been one of Doug's favorite things. And so, in times of crisis, even though a daily task (like cooking) becomes harder, it doesn't go away. Since my diagnosis, there have been many days when I was tired or sick or just used my energy on other tasks and getting a meal on the table for my crew seemed hard.

So many women (and men), but I'll be honest, I think it was mostly women, did some "pinch-hitting" for me and stood in for me. They rang the doorbell and hugged me and walked into our kitchen with meals for our family. All of you chefs might not have known this, but I took your food and served it to my family and in some crazy way it was like I was caring for them and offering them this food. You let me feel like I was still the mom and I was still taking care of my family. When Doug and the girls said, "This is good," I said thank you. Of course, we knew where the meal came from, and we were grateful to all of you with each and every meal. My girls learned how blessed they were and how friends care for each other.

The title of this post came from a song called "How Beautiful The Hands that Serve".

The main idea of the song is that serving others is a true act of Christ-like love.

Again, copyright does not allow sharing the lyrics, but they are worth looking up.

Here is how I hear the song.

How beautiful, the hands that buy, prepare, cook, and bring the food to me and to my family. I am a "daughter" of the earth and the KING and your acts are a beautiful service.

So, to all of you who have prepared a meal for me, I am so grateful and thankful and BLESSED by your act of service.

It is almost 2:00 p.m., and I am happy to say I had my 9th treatment of Taxol today. That leaves three to go. One of the strongest ladies I know, Ms. RaeAnn, went with me. We laughed, talked and she fetched me a blanket and water and a pillow. After we were done, she drove me to Kreger's

Bakery (a hometown tradition) and got me a donut. Doug is watching my diet like a mother hen, so don't worry, Doug, it is only one and I will be diligent with my food choices. It was SO GOOD, THOUGH. It was a cream filled chocolate frosted donut and I savored every single bite!

Reflection

Dang-that food was a real blessing during that treatment. We try to do that for people now whenever we can to pay it forward. Even the girls have gotten into it, and sometimes ask me to make a meal for someone who is sick or sad or struggling. I like that in them. I like to do some bulk cooking sometimes and I have two favorite recipes for mass production-Chicken Divine Casserole and Chicken Pot Pie. The Chicken Divine Casserole is from a church cookbook, the St. Paul Lutheran Church from my home church in Iowa. Our youth group sold these cookbooks for $10.00 each for a fundraiser a LONG time ago.

Here goes—super easy-not GF (gluten-free), DF (dairy-free) or vegan, but really good if you are not following a specific diet. This is comfort food in its truest form. (I tried not to eat too much comfort food when I was going through treatment, but every once in a while I indulged.)

Chicken Breasts (as many as you want)

Swiss Cheese Slices (one for each chicken breast)

Cream of Chicken Soup (for each can, dilute with ½ a can of water)

Butter and Pepperidge Farm Stuffing Mix (1 stick of butter for each three cups of stuffing mix-one package has six cups of stuffing mix)

Basically, you place as many chicken breasts as you want in a 9x13 or 8x8 pan. If you are cooking in bulk, you can use the aluminum disposable pans from Sam's Club or Costco or any grocery store. Cover each chicken breast with a piece of sliced swiss cheese. Then, pour the cream of chicken soup mixture over your chicken and cheese. Again, I usually cook in bulk, so I mix two large cans of soup with one can of water and pour the mixture over. Finally, I add my crumb topping. You can add as much or as little as you like. I usually melt two sticks of butter and add one bag of stuffing mix.

That should be enough for two 9x13 pans. Lastly, cover with foil. If you are making a lot, they freeze beautifully. Just remind the recipient to bake covered with foil or the top will burn.

My second favorite comfort food is Chicken Pot Pie. I got this recipe from my Mom who got it from her friend, Barb, who got it from *Taste of Home* magazine.

Ingredients

2 cups diced peeled potatoes

1-3/4 cups sliced carrots

1 cup butter, cubed

2/3 cup chopped onion

1 cup all-purpose flour

1-3/4 teaspoons salt

1 teaspoon dried thyme

3/4 teaspoon pepper

3 cups chicken broth

1-1/2 cups whole milk

4 cups cubed cooked chicken

1 cup frozen peas

1 cup frozen corn

4 sheets refrigerated pie crust

Preheat the oven to 425°. Place potatoes and carrots in a large saucepan; add water to cover. Bring to a boil. Reduce heat; cook, covered, 8-10 minutes or until crisp-tender; drain.

In a large skillet, heat butter over medium-high heat. Add onion; cook and stir until tender. Stir in flour and seasonings until blended. Gradually stir in broth and milk. Bring to a boil, stirring constantly; cook and stir for 2 minutes or until thickened. Stir in chicken, peas, corn and potato mixture; remove from heat.

Unroll a pie crust into each of two 9-in. pie plates; trim even with rims. Add chicken mixture. Unroll remaining crusts; place over filling. Trim, seal and flute edges. Cut slits in tops.

Bake for 35-40 minutes or until the crust is lightly browned. Let stand 15 minutes before cutting.

Freeze option: Cover and freeze unbaked pies. To use, remove from the freezer 30 minutes before baking (do not thaw). Preheat the oven to 425°. Place pies on baking sheets; cover edges loosely with foil. Bake for 30 minutes. Reduce oven setting to 350°; bake 70-80 minutes longer or until crust is golden brown and a thermometer inserted in center reads 165°.

This is another recipe that is great for making in bulk. We usually triple and we can get about eight pot pies. I buy frozen pie crusts and then buy the refrigerated baking sheets to cover the top of the crusts. I usually use the stretchy gallon bags for freezing.

I will be honest, as I said before, I tried not to eat a lot of comfort food when I was going through treatment. I realize that it might be a bit hypocritical of me to share comfort food recipes here, but many people are dealing with heartache that is not related to a health concern. For things· like new babies or mental health struggles or sadness related to death, I think comfort food is an expression of love. If I know people are following a specific diet, I respect that and offer up whatever the individual or family wants. Also, some cancer patients don't follow a certain diet or change the way they are eating, and that's OK.

That said, as far as food goes, cancer does make many patients question what they are putting into their bodies. I did drastically change my diet and it wasn't hard at all because I was scared. I gave up sugar and Diet Coke and most junk food immediately. Of course, as time passed, I let go of a lot of these restrictions, but now I shoot for a low sugar, quality protein, lots of veggies and fruit plan. Do I think I got cancer from being overweight? Probably not, but I don't know. I have met a lot of women who are awfully thin and who got breast cancer. Still, I don't think it helps anything to be overweight. I guess I see it this way. I am going to try to do everything I can to prevent a recurrence of breast cancer or a new cancer diagnosis. If I suffer one of these things and I am at the right BMI, at least I know I did what I could do. I did what was in my circle of influence. As I write, I am still not at a healthy BMI, but I am trying, I really am.

Doug was also pretty concerned about my diet during my treatment. I fasted 24 hours before each chemotherapy treatment. My oncologist did not recommend or discourage the fasting. Doug found evidence that supported it, but again, this is something you have to research and decide whether or not you feel this would be beneficial to you.

I also took a number of supplements: Turkey Tail, a baby aspirin, Vitamin D, zinc, and melatonin. In addition, once treatment was over, I started a regimen with an organization called Care Oncology Clinic-COC. This is a brief description from the COC website.

What is Care Oncology?

Care Oncology Clinics prescribe a repurposed combination of existing, licensed medications which are used to treat conditions other than cancer. This standard of practice is known as off-label use. Research suggests that these drugs may complement and enhance the effect of traditional, standard-of-care cancer therapies.

I started this protocol right when I finished up the oral chemo I did for six months following surgery. I am planning to do it for three years total, and then I will re-evaluate. The meds cost about $50/month which is out of pocket. I also have a Zoom consultation about once every four months which is about $300. So, the total monthly cost of this protocol is $125/month and none of this is covered by insurance. Again, I know that not all patients can afford this and/or not all patients would try something that is basically "alternative" or "experimental".

I am on one other protocol, but I am not going to discuss it here. Perhaps anyone reading this is asking a few questions: Why are you still "treating yourself" if you are "cured"?

Before facing a cancer diagnosis, I thought or believed that there was a scan or a blood test, or some way to tell if a patient was cancer free. Now, I realize that a better way to describe a patient's cancer status is NED, or NO EVIDENCE OF DISEASE. Many times, testing can only identify cancer when it has grown enough to be identified. For example, my father-in-law declared himself cancer free when he finished his first round of chemo for lung cancer and the PET scan did not detect any cancer in his body. Unfortunately, there was cancer there, it just wasn't able to be identified by the means of testing available at the time. Just months later, we learned that the cancer had spread to his brain. He received radiation and did live longer. In my case, I was/am operating under the assumption that there were/are still some breast cancer cells floating around and I wanted/want to do everything I could do/can do to ward them off. A recurrence could be local, but in a more difficult case scenario, a recurrence could be metastatic. Metastatic cancer cannot be cured, and like most metastatic cancers, metastatic triple negative breast cancer is not a good prognosis.

Why would you seek out alternative treatments? Why wouldn't you just be satisfied with what your oncologist(s)/surgeons tell you to do? I cannot emphasize enough how much I respect the providers who cared and still care for me. They are individuals who have devoted their lives to understanding and treating cancer, and they know infinitely more than I know. That said, healthcare in the United States and treatment protocols are highly regulated and governed. Providers will, for the most part, offer treatment that has been studied and gone through many trials. And, that is VERY IMPORTANT AND NECESSARY AND OFFERS THE BEST CHANCE AT A CURE AND/OR LONGER SURVIVAL. Still, there are folks who are adding complementary treatments to standard treatment protocols and finding success. This requires a lot of reading and researching and a bit of faith and sometimes a bit of money (but not always). Some of the things I did, like fasting before chemo and exercising regularly during chemo did not cost anything. Adding a baby aspirin to my daily regimen costs pennies. I was very blessed because I had a husband who could sift through the "junk" science and the real science and make sense of it for me. My point here is that you do not need to be completely passive about your treatment. You may find some things you can add to your regimen that may help fight cancer.

TO BOOB OR NOT TO BOOB, THAT IS THE QUESTION

JOURNAL ENTRY BY HEIDI EDWARDS
NOVEMBER 13, 2017

To be or not to be: that is the question. Hamlet

To boob or not to boob: that is the question. Heidi

I am writing this from the "Infusion Room" at the Cancer Center. My sweet Doug and I got here at about ten this morning. (He had the day off, and what better place to spend it. Insert sarcasm here.) I got my blood drawn at about 10:15 a.m., and then we saw Dr. Anand. I didn't expect to see him this week as I saw him last week, but after the CNA weighed me and took my temperature, she took me to an exam room. I think the visit may have been because I was at Mayo last Wednesday (11/8) and Dr. Anand wanted to discuss that visit with me. Chatting with him was helpful, and now I am waiting for the nurses to start the weekly Taxol treatment. That will be number 10 of 12 treatments!!

The appointments at Mayo were set-up last July, and part of me was surprised when November 8th came so quickly. It seems like I have been doing the "whole cancer thing" for a long time now. After being at Mayo, my thoughts and actions have turned from chemotherapy to surgery. My brain has shifted gears. The big challenge for me right now is deciding what to do surgically.

The positive (and tricky) part is that I have a choice about what to do. I am glad I have a choice, but choices are also tricky because the ball is in your hands and the choices become more laden with responsibility. One surgical option is a lumpectomy, a procedure where the surgeon just removes any remaining tumor (hopefully there is none) and the tumor bed around the tumor. Pathology is involved to make sure that the margins are clear and that no cancerous cells are left behind. Of course, nothing is guaranteed, but that's the goal.

The other option(s) are a unilateral (one breast) mastectomy or a bilateral (both breasts) mastectomy. This option begets the reconstruction option. If I decide on a mastectomy (of either sort) and opt for reconstruction, I could have implants or the plastic surgeon could create breasts from my tummy fat or from the muscle in my back. The first option (with implants) is the least invasive, and the second two options are BIG surgeries—it takes around 12 hours to create new breasts from the tummy fat or back muscle. With implant based reconstruction, an expander is placed at the time of surgery. The expander is swapped out with the permanent implant a few months later in the "exchange" surgery. The second options (from a person's own fat/muscle) are done several months after the initial mastectomy. Also, with any reconstruction option, there is little to no sensation in the new "breasts". I would like to note that there are also patients who choose to have a mastectomy and choose not to have any reconstruction. I have heard this referred to as "going flat".

What to do? What to do? What to do?

Statistically, the long term survival rates are the same with lumpectomy and radiation versus mastectomy alone. So, it really comes down to personal preference. The biggest benefit to mastectomy is emotional peace of mind. Certainly, the risk of a new breast cancer developing is very small and the possibility of recurrence in the affected breast is slightly smaller with a mastectomy than with a lumpectomy. That said, any spreading of the cancer to other body parts cannot be prevented by a mastectomy. Plus, a mastectomy is a bigger surgery with a longer recovery time. If reconstruction is involved, the healing time is even longer.

The biggest benefit to a lumpectomy is that YOU STILL HAVE YOUR OWN BREASTS and you still have sensation in your breasts. Also, obviously, the recovery time is shorter, and usually, there is no or less reconstruction involved. The downside is mostly emotional/psychological in that some women worry about the cancer returning or remaining in the affected breast. There is also worry about a new cancer developing. Dr. Anand told me the risk of that is .05% a year with the risk accumulating each year. (In other words, in 30 years, I would have a 15% risk of breast cancer.) Finally, a patient will almost always do radiation with lumpectomy. In my case, radiation would probably mean five weeks of treatment each day from Monday to Friday. Radiation brings its own set of concerns. IF I have a mastectomy and IF the cancer has not spread to any lymph nodes, I might be able to avoid radiation.

My surgery is set-up for December 27th. I do need to come to Mayo the day before for an injection of a dye to check my lymph nodes at the time of surgery. I have a few weeks to decide what to do, and I am praying for clear guidance on this. In the end, though, I realize that I am trying to make a decision based on events I have no control over. If I knew that I would have a future recurrence or that I would have a new cancer develop in my breast, of course I would do a mastectomy (with implant based reconstruction). If I knew that would never be an issue, I would opt for the lumpectomy.

There is just this part of me that believes the more radical option (mastectomy) would be more preventative and that a lumpectomy is just too "good to be true". I know that logically this is not correct. The first breast surgeon I met with said that if there was a conveyor belt to take newly diagnosed patients from her office to the operating room for a bilateral mastectomy, almost all patients would hop on and have her "cut them off". She told me (way back in July) to make this decision not only based on emotion, but on logic.

And so............I am trying to do that. That said, I am praying for guidance and praying that I will have peace in whatever choice I make.

It is now 8:30 p.m. on Monday night. Treatment went well, and I was so happy to have Doug by my side, the place he has been since the moment breast cancer came into our lives.

Reflection

In the initial stages of diagnosis, I did meet with the surgeon and even a plastic surgeon, but I couldn't really even think about surgery because I was just wrapping my head around chemotherapy. If I were in charge of coordinating breast cancer care for patients, I think I would offer them two options at the beginning of their cancer journey.

Option One-Meet with all the specialists that might be involved in your care including a radiation oncologist, a general surgeon, and a plastic surgeon. Note—A cancer patient meets with his or her oncologist regularly throughout the whole journey and after active treatment is completed. (In some cases, a person is always in "active" treatment.)

Option Two-After meeting with your oncologist and deciding on your plan of care, meet only with the specialists that are relevant at that time.

I would have chosen Option Two. I met with all the specialists right away, but it was overwhelming for me and I never even ended up having radiation. For a while, I considered not having reconstruction, but in the end, I did.

I agonized over the surgical decision for a good couple of weeks. Dr. Anand encouraged me to do a lumpectomy, and I think his rationale was very logical and reasonable. The reason I ended up having a mastectomy was largely emotional, and I acknowledge that. I think I made the right decision, though, because I do not have any regrets four years later. The only regret I have is that I have very little sensation in my breasts. That is fine, though, totally fine. I decided to do the "easiest" form of reconstruction, implant based reconstruction. I did not want to go through another big surgery post-mastectomy. Again, I acknowledge that the reconstruction piece of breast cancer is very, very personal and there is no one size fits all approach. Each patient must sift through the information available and his or her emotions, make a choice, and try not to look back and second guess her (or his) choice.

THE CANCER CONNECTION

JOURNAL ENTRY BY HEIDI EDWARDS
NOVEMBER 20, 2017

I met Agnes (not her real name) at the Cancer Center. I don't know when exactly we met, but it was early on in my treatment. I also didn't know her age, but I would guess she was in her 70's. It is a bit harder to guess someone's age when they don't have hair. She is a petite woman, and her clothes have looked looser every time I see her. I know that Agnes has lung cancer. Week after week, I would see her and week after week she did not look well. One week she needed a blood transfusion, and there was a week when she could not get her chemo because she was not well enough. Each week we would chat and squeeze each other's hands (hers were always cold) and check in with each other. One week I brought her a little candle. Recently, I was sitting in a recliner in the infusion room, getting my Taxol, when Agnes walked in. "I had a scan today, and the doctor can't see anything," she said. "The doctor is giving me four weeks off," she said, and I watched the tears run down her face. "I wanted to tell you my good news. I also want to wish you good luck and thank you again for the candle you gave me. I burn it just a little every night." She came over, bent over me, and hugged me, and then she was gone. When she left, I started crying because I was so happy for her and because I wanted her to be OK.

Cancer has connected me to others, too.

Recently, a woman from my church was also diagnosed with cancer. She has children fairly close to the ages of my children. I knew her, but since her diagnosis we have shared many texts and compared notes as we are both receiving Taxol (she has infusions of another drug as well). She sent me a pic of herself when she shaved her head and I told her she looked beautiful. (She really did look beautiful.) We talk about sleep and what to eat and other "cancer stuff".

Another breast cancer patient (the sister-in-law of a friend) who has never even met me, heard from her sister-in-law about me and sent me a big box of goodies. When I called her to thank her, we talked for almost an hour about her diagnosis and treatment and life post breast cancer. She sent me a picture of herself about a week later via text. I sent her a text back and told her she looked so strong and healthy and happy.

There is also the teenage girl with blood cancer I wrote about in a post from August. I was at a restaurant in the Dells with my college friends when a Dad from the table next to me bent over and asked if I was in treatment. When I said yes, he said his daughter had just finished treatment. He told me his daughter wanted to hug me and asked me if that would be OK. When I said yes, she came over and we melted into each other. Her heart opened up, my heart opened up and we connected in a way that only two people who have both had cancer and chemo could connect. When she and her family left, I had to go to the bathroom and collect myself. I pray and hope that girl is back in high school and doing what high school kids should be doing. (They should not be getting chemo.)

And there are others who have connected with me.........

Another woman who also had thyroid and breast cancer who contacted me via email to offer support

My neighbors (both men) with cancer who encourage me every time they see me

The women at the Eye Clinic (where Doug works) who have battled breast cancer and other forms of cancer and who have reached out with cards and offers to talk "at any time"

A relative of my aunt's who sent me peppermint oil to help with nausea even though she had never met me (she is currently battling breast cancer as well)—*She passed away from breast cancer since my original post.*

A dental hygienist at our dental office who met me for coffee to mull over surgical options (another breast cancer survivor)

The couple from our church who stopped at our house one afternoon with flowers, a gift, and a beautiful card with a message of support (the woman is a breast cancer survivor)

MM—a young breast cancer survivor, just starting her married life when she was diagnosed

AP—a woman in her early 30's in Seattle who also dealt with triple negative breast cancer, we connected through friends

KR-a young mom of two kiddos whose own mother-in-law lost her battle with cancer while KR was going through treatment

OB-GYN Nurse/SK—another mom of four kids-we connected through a woman in my Book Club, we met at a diner once and her family came over for a meal once

When these patients and survivors hug me or hold my hand or in some cases, talk or text, I know they UNDERSTAND. I see it in their eyes and hear it in their voices and sometimes, we share tears. Some of these people are much farther in their cancer journeys, and their lives and stories are hopeful and healing. I am ahead of some of these other patients in my walk. I pray that I can offer this hope to others in the future, that I can help people feel less alone in this journey.

Happy note........

I COMPLETED MY 11TH TAXOL TREATMENT TODAY. I ONLY HAVE ONE LEFT. Stacy sat with me and we talked and met another patient, an 84-year-old woman who told me I had a beautiful face and made my day. We treated ourselves to some peppermints before we left the Cancer Center. When I got home, my friend Kim brought over spaghetti and meatballs for dinner. I picked up the twins and we went to Kreger's for a donut (chemo day treat). Now I am sitting with Maves (nickname for Avery), watching American Pickers, and snuggling. If that isn't a good day, I don't know what is!

Reflection

I can't even remember all the names now of people I met just because of cancer. I should have kept track of them. These connections were and still are a hidden blessing. I am still meeting people because of cancer—people I never would have met if I had not had cancer.

I hate cheesiness, and some of this sounds really cheesy, but the connections and bonds made over cancer are immediate. Some of these survivors I still talk to, but most of them I don't. That is a good thing because we have moved on with our lives. We are OK. We don't need each other anymore, but there was this special period in time and space when our paths crossed and we did life together. All of these people will always be very important to me.

PART ONE DONE

JOURNAL ENTRY BY HEIDI EDWARDS
NOVEMBER 28, 2017

I was hoping to get this update posted yesterday, but my last chemo wasn't until 2:30, so I had the whole morning to WAIT. I did get some stuff done around the house as last week was a bit of traveling and then a lot of mess-making.

We started our Thanksgiving holiday by leaving Wednesday morning and driving to Adair, Iowa, where my younger brother, Cory, his wife, Jody, and their three kids live. They welcomed us with open arms, fed us, and gave us comfy beds to sleep in. On Thursday, my Mom and Dad and my other brother, Jason, who is cognitively and physically challenged, arrived as well. My brother and sister-in-law also graciously invited Doug's brother, his wife, and their three kids and they made the trek from Sioux City, Iowa. The final guests were Jody's parents, Jim and Rita. All I can say is..............BEST. THANKSGIVING. EVER! Thanks to Jody, Jody's mom, and my Mom, the food was AMAZING. (I did not do anything!) After lunch, my brother loaded up three 4-wheelers and we went out to his "farm", a piece of land he has developed into a playground. There is a little cabin, a covered pavilion, a pond, and trails for the 4-wheelers. I sat under the pavilion and Doug took me for a 4-wheeler ride. On Friday afternoon, we left and headed back to Wisconsin. Saturday and Sunday we were at home making messes.

Moving on...........

Yesterday I finished my twenty-week chemo journey. My mom and dad came up on Sunday evening. They were here for the first treatment, and they wanted to be here for the last. My mom gave me some silver, sparkly earrings and a poem she had written for me. My dad went to treatment with me while my mom stayed at home to help with a little "surprise".

The treatment was happily uneventful. Ms. Amy stopped by the infusion room with a "trophy" she made for me, a little bottle of champagne, and some cupcakes. Once the oncology nurse unhooked me, Amy pushed me around on a roller chair for a victory lap. I got some good love from the other patients. We also pulled off the final picture of my doctor's head from my "chemo crown". Then, even though we could have left, we stayed and talked for 15 minutes.

Dad and I were home by about 4:40 or so. When we opened the door, it was quiet and the lights were dim. Within seconds, out popped Lauren and Ave, Sophia (one of my "adopted" daughters—her sis, Charlotte, couldn't be there) and my Mom. A group of beautiful, amazing, and very loving ladies came in and decorated the house with balloons and pictures and a string of paper bras. They left cards and donuts (from Kreger's) and pink ribbon tattoos. I felt loved beyond measure. My mom had been in on the surprise, too, and kept it all a secret.

We ate a wonderful meal brought over by Ms. Jill and then we celebrated birthdays. Mom's is on the 29th and G's is on the 8th. Then we all collapsed in the living room and it was good.

I am taking a little liberty with the Bible verse below, but I think God would be OK with that. Praise the Lord (for bringing me through chemo)! Give thanks to the Lord, for he is good (in giving me friends and family to walk beside me and doctors to care for me)! His faithful love endures forever (even in the next step of breast cancer). Psalm 106:1

Reflection

When I read some of these posts now, I feel like they might come off as a little Pollyannaish. Maybe I can look back on this time now in an optimistic way because I survived, and I have had a positive outcome. I know that the cancer could come back at some time; I understand that, but I have been really lucky and right now the future looks really hopeful for me. One thing that I did struggle with at the end of chemo was that there was a sense of celebration around finishing twenty weeks of infusions, but I didn't really feel like I could celebrate. I knew that I had surgery ahead and reconstruction and maybe radiation. I knew that my prognosis was heavily dependent on what the pathology post-surgery showed. I wanted to be really happy, but I couldn't really allow myself to let my guard down. I did celebrate, but it was a half-hearted celebration.

TRIBUTE TO DOUG

JOURNAL ENTRY BY HEIDI EDWARDS
DECEMBER 4, 2017

It is Monday, December 4th, and I DON'T HAVE CHEMO TODAY. Today is very gray and rainy. We have enjoyed an uncommon week of gorgeous, warm, sunny weather here in the Northwoods, so I really cannot complain. Doug's taxi service left about 30 minutes ago with the three girls. He picks up two more "passengers" before making a stop at the middle school and then the high school. Avery was having a mini breakdown because she "forgot" about some ELA homework (English Language Arts). Grace was trying to balance her twenty pound backpack (literally), workout bag, and coffee as she left. Lauren was interrogating us all and trying to figure out "who ate the peppermints from her cubby that she got after helping at children's church yesterday?" I will be honest, I ate one, but that's all. When they left, the house went from a decibel level of 10 to 1 in a second. I know that I only witnessed the end of the chaos this morning as I woke up just in time (6:55 a.m.) to say goodbye. On days when he is in town, Doug takes the girls and I sleep until I wake up. On days when he is out of town, I get up, but even then I don't usually get up until about 6:30, in time to leave the house at seven for school drop-off. God bless that sweet, sweet man! (He called me at about eight this morning from a clinic phone telling me that he forgot his cell phone and that he was wearing two different shoes. He thought it was because the "girls got him a little bit riled up".) I told him I would bring a matching shoe and his cell phone to him.

When you get married, there is absolutely no way you can anticipate what life will bring. There is also absolutely no way you can anticipate how your partner will react to what life brings.

From the day I was diagnosed, Doug was ON IT. Within an hour of "THE CALL" on a Wednesday, he was on the phone reaching out to a colleague at Mayo for help in being seen there. And, on Friday, we were at Mayo. He rearranged his schedule to be with me that day, and a day the following week.

He quickly started ordering books on Amazon and books with titles like *Keto for Cancer, Tripping over the Truth, Surviving Triple Negative Breast Cancer*, and *The Breast Cancer Husband* started arriving at our house. He found the researchers who were at the forefront of research in triple negative breast cancer and even emailed one poor woman over and over and over until she responded to him. He did make a donation to her research. :) He joined Facebook groups and talked to an MD in Florida who adds complementary medicine to traditional oncology treatments. Under the advice of this physician, and with the blessing of my oncologist in Wausau, Doug started me on a regimen of some supplements.

While I am not as strict as I should be, I have changed my diet in response to cancer. I try to avoid gluten and most dairy (not cheese). I try to limit my carbs and sugar. I am eating broccoli sprouts as often as I can. (We tried sprouting our own, but that turned out to be a time consuming, stinky mess.) Initially, I just really couldn't eat because I was so upset, but as I got my appetite back, Doug encouraged me to eat differently. He did this by sending me text after text after text with links discussing the role of diet in fighting certain types of cancer and the importance of trying to get to a more appropriate BMI.

That boy has also pulled me off the sofa or recliner and got me walking. There was a day after the AC chemo when Doug came home and found me in our darkened bedroom, in the recliner, covered with blankets. I was a hot mess. I tried to complain to him. He did not say anything. He just got me my shoes, watched me put them on, grabbed my hand, and took me for a walk. We mostly walk up Rib Mountain, but we also love Sunnyvale and the Quarry and our neighborhood. He bought me a heart rate monitor that I don't wear. I am also doing some training with Ms. Sarah, a wonderful friend who also happens to be a trainer.

He has cried with me, but mostly he has helped me recognize that I have a lot of power in this situation. I can eat right and exercise and be active and social and keep living. I can choose to wrap my identity around having breast cancer or I can wrap my identity around who I still am and how cancer will change me for the better. I can sit in a recliner in a dark room and cry or get up and walk and talk and make plans and do all the things I love.

So, when I married Doug 21 years ago (he was only 22 and I was only 23), I knew he was special, but his love and faithfulness and perseverance have turned out to be beyond anything I could have hoped for.

On a side note, I will go to Mayo next week for a bit of testing. I have decided to have a double mastectomy with implant-based reconstruction. Surgery is scheduled for December 27th.

Reflection

On Tuesday, May 18th, 2021, Doug and I celebrated 25 years of marriage. I actually remember my parents 25th. We didn't have Grace until we were almost 30 and we had the twins at 33, so we had almost seven years of marriage before kids. My parents had their children at a younger age, so my siblings and I were older at my parent's 25th. We had a little party in their front yard with cake and food. Doug's parents even came from Sioux City for the event, and my Mom and Dad gave up their bedroom (for my in-laws) for the weekend. I still remember how much fun my father-in-law had, and talked about it for years. It was a beautiful June day when we celebrated.

Back to Doug, though...... He has been a good life partner, the best really, and I hope that I never have to live without him. I know that lots of people have to go through a cancer diagnosis and treatment without a partner, and I can only imagine the additional struggle that is. That said, one of the biggest things cancer clarified for me is that there are a whole host of people who are the hands and feet of Jesus and who will be there. Those people (the hands and feet of Jesus) might just need to be asked, but they will be there and stand in the gap. I would do that for someone, and I hope and pray that I already have.

AM I REALLY SICK?

JOURNAL ENTRY BY HEIDI EDWARDS
DECEMBER 11, 2017

One of the weirdest things about this whole deal is the fact that when I was diagnosed, I didn't FEEL sick at all. In fact, I felt absolutely FINE. Once chemo started, I felt sick, but the sickness and fatigue came and went in waves.

Today is my two-week anniversary of finishing chemo, and I am feeling stronger every day. Yesterday, after gorging ourselves at a "Santa Brunch", we all walked up the hill (Rib Mountain). Lauren kind of "whined" up the hill, but, in fairness, she does have a cold. It was easier than it had been the week before. My legs felt stronger and I really wasn't out of breath. Grace looped her arm through mine and we climbed together.

It was the end of a FUN and BUSY weekend. G turned 15 on Friday and we celebrated her actual birthday with dinner at Chang Garden with some family friends. On Saturday, Grace had a little party with some of her buddies at a place called U Paint and Party. This is a business where the owner/artist leads a group as they paint a pre-picked piece of art. In this case, the piece of art was the head of a cow. G was worried the girls wouldn't like it, but they looked pretty darn happy to me as they painted their cow faces and enjoyed mocktails. We (just Doug and I) ended our Saturday with dinner at some friends' house. G made boiled eggs and boiled carrots for herself and her sisters. (The boiled eggs went over pretty well- the boiled carrots not so much.) Still, my baby is developing some basics in the kitchen. She would make my middle-school home economics teacher, Mrs. Delaney, proud.

And so, by the time Sunday rolled around, I was tired, but who wouldn't be? Really?

During the weekend, there were times that I completely forgot that I had cancer. It doesn't really seem REAL right now. I am in this weird in-between place. Chemo finished on 11/27 and surgery is 12/27. Since I am not in active treatment, I catch myself wondering if it is OK to be myself again, to forget about this. I can't really forget though, because today I find myself at Mayo again. I was blessed enough to come down today with a kind friend whose husband is also doctoring here for a few days. I am going to meet with the general surgeon, the plastic surgeon, and have some imaging done. Doug will join me for part of the time, and I am enjoying a little time alone as well. Too bad you have to get breast cancer to have a little holiday all by yourself. Ha! Ha! Ha! And so, I know it is real, but there are moments when breast cancer still seems unreal.

I talked to Doug when I got here, and he asked me if I was OK or if being here was making me scared. I answered him truthfully when I said I just want to be done. I want to be well. I want to let my guard down, but I can't really relax because this big thing is hanging over me.

That's just life though. Life is full of these weird juxtapositions that you just have to kind of work through. The hard part is living in the in-between place.

I am OK though. I have good doctors, good support, a good plan, the prospect of a very good outcome, and a good FATHER—a heavenly one. You just gotta keep perspective.

Reflections

That birthday party was a lot of fun, it really was. It was also expensive, and one of Grace's best parties ever. I did it because I wondered if it might be the last birthday party I got to celebrate with her. It sounds morbid, and I never told anyone that, but that is the truth. We had a lot of fun; we did the same thing for the girls when they turned 12 in April. I think Grace gave her cow to my brother, and Lauren and Avery's cows are hanging in the cabin now. We catered in Qdoba and ended up with a whole bunch of extra tortilla chips that we munched on for days. Grace was gifted with a lot of candles and socks and bath bombs. Bath bombs were really popular there for a while. I don't see them as much now, but for a while there were lots of baths and bath bombs happening at our house.

UPDATE FROM MAYO

Journal Entry by Heidi Edwards
December 18, 2017

Last week I spent a few days at Mayo Clinic (dubbed World Famous Mayo Clinic or WFMC by Doug), in preparation for my upcoming surgery. As I mentioned earlier, it is honestly kind of like the Disney World of medicine, but in a serene, dignified sort of way. It is almost like a cathedral in some areas, and even though there are thousands of people passing through the clinic every day, it is never really loud or chaotic. Every patient has a printed "visit itinerary" and as you visit each stop, the receptionist scans the barcode at the bottom of your itinerary to check you in. At each doctor appointment, you receive a beeper that buzzes when the provider is ready for you.

Doug and I lived in Rochester for three years while he did his oph-thalmology residency. Like many residencies, it provided him with the training he needed to begin practicing medicine, but it was also fairly pain-ful. He is grateful for the solid education he received, but he wouldn't want to do it again. When I come to Mayo, I am grateful, but I always leave a bit fearful as well. The doctors here are certainly optimistic, but they are more guarded and cautious and careful about what they say.

The visit to Mayo was very positive, though. I had an MRI, mam-mogram, and ultrasound. All three exams showed that the tumor was considerably smaller. Also, it is possible that part of what is remaining is actually scar tissue or DCIS, a lower-grade kind of cancer that may not even respond to chemo. I met my surgeon, a woman in her 50's (I guess), whose surgical focus is only on breast disease/breast cancer. She was kind and told me she would take good care of me. I also met the reconstructive surgeon. She was fairly easy-going and we even shared a few laughs.

I need to be at Mayo on the 26th to have a small radioactive marker placed in the lesion. This will help the surgeon in removing the lesion a.k.a. tumor and the area around the lesion. I also need to have a dye injected in my breast to test the lymph nodes and make sure the cancer has not moved to the nodes. I will also see an OB/GYN that day to discuss removing my ovaries (later in 2018).

On the day of surgery, the breast surgeon will remove my breasts, but leave enough skin to create "new breasts". Unfortunately, because my breasts are too droopy, the nipples cannot be spared. (I was not at all offended when both the surgeons told me my breasts were droopy; in the whole scheme of things, it was kind of funny.) Then, before the reconstructive surgeon begins, pathology will make sure all the margins are clear. This could be a relatively quick process OR it could take a bit. (Either way, I will be asleep.) Then, the reconstructive surgeon, Dr. Le, will begin. Dr. Le will place two temporary expanders under my chest muscles and inflate them a bit with saline. Then, she will sew everything back up, and I will have "new" breasts. (They will not be their permanent size.)

I will have a drain on each side that will stay in for one to two weeks. The expanders will have a port; at each visit to the plastic surgeon, a bit more saline will be injected. If I need radiation, the process will be a bit slower. If not, it will be a bit quicker. Once radiation is complete (if needed) and the expanders have stretched the skin to the size I want, there will be an exchange surgery. At this time, the expanders will come out and the new permanent implants will go in. As a final step, I am thinking about nipple tattoos; that is much later though.

Honestly, I am tired just thinking about it, but the good news is that it doesn't happen in one day; it will be a process. In the interim, life will just keep moving and this will just be one part of my life, not my whole life.

Speaking of other great parts of my life, we had a good weekend. Doug was on-call and he worked a lot this weekend. Most of his Saturday was spent taking care of eyes. The girls and I whooped it up while he was working. On Saturday night, all three of the girls dressed up Avery's guinea pigs in little Christmas outfits from PetSmart and did a photoshoot. It made me SO HAPPY to see the pictures. On Sunday, Ave went out to the barn with her "horse mama and horse sister" (a wonderful woman and her daughter who have graciously been taking Ave with them when they go) and Lauren made gingerbread men. She has been asking to do this all week, and she was finally able. I was kind of holding out because anyway you cut it, an 11-year-old baker is a pretty messy baker. While L was baking, Grace did a photo shoot with me as her model. She has been taking pictures of her friends for quite a while, and wanted to take pics of me. So, she did my make-up and I posed (if you can call it that). Who knew modeling was such hard work?

It's Monday night now; I am one day closer to surgery, and I am grateful for that. For all you prayer warriors out there, I have a few specific requests.

1. peace for myself as I wait for the 27th
2. health for myself and my doctors
3. that the doctors use the talents and gifts God has given them
4. a good outcome from the surgery—clean lymph nodes and removal of all the cancer

Reflections

The two weeks before surgery were actually really stressful. I kept worrying that I would get sick or that the surgeon would get sick and I wouldn't be able to have my surgery. I remember trying to help the girls put together little Christmas gifts for their sixth grade teachers and being so short with them. They couldn't decide what they wanted and debated back and forth and I was just like "whatever already, just pick something", but they agonized over every little detail. I was kind of grumpy and just nervous. I didn't know how long I would be out of commission. I labeled the dividers in the silverware drawer in preparation for my "time out". I wrote Little Forks, Big Forks, Knives, Tablespoons, Teaspoons on the wooden Pioneer Woman silverware holder from Wal-Mart. I labeled another drawer divider

Serving Utensils, another Knives/Scissors/and Thermometers. A third was Miscellaneous and the last was Openers. In the girls' dressers, more labels appeared: Leggings, Socks, Underwear, Jeans, T-shirts, Etc. I stocked up on laundry soap, dish detergent, dishwasher detergent, toilet paper, and paper towels. I gave the house a really good cleaning. We moved the recliner from next to the bed to a more open spot. (I had purchased the recliner when I first started chemo.) I moved a small side table next to it, and added a lamp. My friend RaeAnn sent me a post mastectomy shirt that I packed in my suitcase. We also packed a drink that is something like Ensure for post-surgical recovery. Doug had read that it was really supposed to help with healing. I was "nesting" in preparation for a period of being out of commission.

NIGHT BEFORE SURGERY

JOURNAL ENTRY BY HEIDI EDWARDS
DECEMBER 26, 2017

Life has this weird way of bringing us back to places we have already been for different reasons. The patterns of our lives converge and then diverge in ways we can never predict.

Flashback to a little over fifteen years ago—Doug and I were living in Rochester, MN. (It was 15 years ago at the time of the post.) We lived at the Valhalla Condominium Complex where we were some of THE ONLY residents under 65. There was an indoor pool at Valhalla with a big sign posted on the door advising residents "DO NOT SWIM IF YOU HAVE HAD ANY INCIDENCE OF DIARRHEA IN THE LAST 24 HOURS". My dad always got a kick out of that, and still jokes about the seemingly unnecessary warning. Ok, back to early December 2002, a little over a decade and a half ago. Doug and I had been married for six and a half years and we were anxiously expecting Grace. She was due on December 4th, but she was not actually born until December 8th. I remember the week before she was born as a time of uneasy, anxious waiting. Even though I worked until three days before her birth, my mind was always in another place. I knew that my/our life was about to change radically, but there was really nothing I could do to prepare. I just had to wait, and when she was born, our lives DID change radically and I don't know if anything could have really prepared us for the way a baby would change our lives.

This last week has been like that as well. I have been busy, but my mind has always been focused on the upcoming surgery. The girls had school through Friday, and on Saturday we celebrated our family Christmas. On Sunday, we went to church in the morning, took a CHILLY walk around the neighborhood, and drove to Iowa. Monday was a celebration with my family at my Mom and Dad's and a late night drive to Rochester. Today I had some pre-op appointments at Mayo. So, we have been busy, but still, it feels like time is going so slowly. I know my life is going to change, but I don't really know how or to what degree. The main change will be the loss of my breasts, and it is hard to know if that will be a terribly emotional thing for me or if it will bother me less than I imagine. I have talked to and read about women on both ends of the spectrum.

As we drove into downtown Rochester last night, I was struck by the connection between this time in my life and that December in 2002 (albeit in early vs. later December) fifteen years ago. When G was born, it was just Doug and I. Now, here at Mayo again, it is just Doug and I. During both of these times, there has been anxious waiting. Life has brought us back to a place where we lived years ago, but this time we came for a different reason. When we left Rochester the first time, we never looked back. We left Rochester on July 1, 2003 (the day after Doug finished his residency) and did not return until July 7, 2017 (the day I came back for my initial oncology appointment here).

I don't think this convergence and divergence is random or coincidental. I think that it is part of a master plan.

As it turned out, life after Grace was born was better and richer and more meaningful. I have to believe that life post-surgery will be better and richer and more meaningful.

Ok, here's the scoop on tomorrow. I will probably go in for surgery between 7:30-8 a.m. The surgery will take between four and six hours. I will ask Doug to post an update here post-surgery with more information. My mom and dad are taking care of the girls which is a HUGE BLESSING AND RELIEF for us.

Many thanks to all of you for supporting me and reaching out to me and praying for me. Please continue to pray for the health of the doctors and for my health, for peace for me and my family, that God will be glorified in this situation, and that the surgery will remove all the cancer from my body.

Signing off as a daughter of the King—Heidi

Reflection

Doug and I actually came to Rochester the evening of the 25th which was a Monday and Christmas Day. We had come to my parents' house in Iowa the day before (Sunday). The reason for traveling to Iowa was two-fold. First of all, it was nice to celebrate with my family. Secondly, and more importantly, we were planning to have the girls stay with my Mom and Dad for about a week. At the end of the week, my mom and dad planned to bring the girls back up to WI and stay with us for a few weeks to help me get back on my feet. Doug was able to take the Christmas holiday off (thus the reason for having my surgery on December 27th), but he would go back after New Year's. We were only at Mom and Dad's for about 24 hours before leaving for Mayo. We had a quick Christmas which we all tried to enjoy, but the surgery was just hanging over us like a dark cloud. When we left, the little girls were fine, but poor Grace was just a wreck, and her pain and worry felt overwhelming to me. After talking to her and realizing that she really needed to be with us, we arranged for her to catch a ride up to Rochester with my friend, Jodi, who was planning to come up to Rochester the day of surgery and stay for one night. I think Grace just needed to physically be there to see what was happening as it happened in real time. Our trip up to Rochester was uneventful, and I was glad to be alone with Doug and not have to guard any emotions.

Tuesday the 26th was busy. The first appointment was with a radiologist, who used ultrasound to insert a radioactive marker at the sight of the tumor. Next we visited with an OB/GYN, but I don't even remember what we talked about. The last appointment of the day was having the blue dye injected into my breasts. This was on December 26th, mind you, and there were not very many people in the clinic. I think that I was the last patient of the day for the person who did the injection, and it was surreal. Have you ever had the experience where you are repainting and/or replacing the carpet in your house, and because you know that is happening, you let your kiddos have fun on the walls? If you are repainting AND replacing the carpets, you don't worry about paint spilling on the carpets. That is how it was with my breasts. By the end of Tuesday, my left breast had a radioactive marker placed by/in the tumor. Both breasts had lots and lots of blue dye injected in direct spots around my nipples. The spots where the dye was injected were swollen and ugly. Really, though, who cared? The carpet was being replaced and the walls repainted. Those girls were coming off in the a.m., and I had already started disassociating from them.

The night before surgery I couldn't really eat. I don't mean because of doctor's orders, I mean just because I was anxious. (I think the doctor had told me to stop eating at eight and to stop drinking at midnight.) I had brought some Honey Roasted Girl Scout Nuts with me from Iowa and I remember sitting by the hotel pool eating them while waiting for our laundry to finish drying. I figured there was no reason for Doug to have to pack up two days of dirty laundry, so I washed and dried the clothes from Monday and Tuesday. I also packed up all of our stuff and packed what I wanted Doug to bring to the hospital. We were staying at a hotel that was attached to the hospital which made it so convenient for both of us, and Doug planned to bring my bag up to the room after surgery.

The night before surgery, in addition to not really eating, I couldn't really sleep, but I knew that it didn't matter because I would basically be sleeping all day the next day and hopefully the next and lots of days after. I took a shower with Hibiclens. (I still remember the name Hibiclens.) The surgeon had given it to me at my appointment in mid-December. I washed my hair and brushed my teeth. I dozed on and off all night, just waiting for the morning to come. One of Doug's superpowers is that he can sleep through anything. I listened to him alternate in and out of snoring. I played on my phone and watched as the clock on the bedside table moved from two to three to four to finally five a.m. The alarm went off on that clock, then my phone, and finally Doug's phone. The last reminder to wake up came in the form of a wake-up call from the front desk. I guess we were worried we would oversleep and miss the surgery?

I got up first and took another shower with Hibiclens. I brushed my teeth carefully, without swallowing any water. I turned on the TV while Doug showered and by 5:40 we were headed down the hallway of the hotel. We walked to where the hotel met the Galleria, an indoor shopping center with a few restaurants. Nothing was open at that hour, and the only people we saw were other patients with their families. As we kept walking and entered the actual clinic, we noticed a few more people—doctors, nurses, maintenance staff. We kept walking until we were in Methodist Hospital, one of two hospitals at Mayo in Rochester. Once we got to the spot where we were supposed to check in, we waited for the first of many "waits" that morning. We were one of three or four parties in line and the check-in process was quick and efficient. I received a bracelet with my name, my clinic number, and my date of birth. From there, we headed to an elevator up to another check-in station at what was more like a nurse's station.

A nurse's aide escorted me to a small room with a recliner and another chair. I changed into a hospital gown and put all my clothes into an apparel bag. I was given a gown that hooked up to warm forced air to keep me warm and that made me look like the Michelin tire man. A medical assistant brought a huge scale to weigh me and an RN came and asked lots and lots of questions about any meds I was taking, any past reactions to anesthesia, and questions about my medical history. I played on my phone for a while and then got distracted and chatted with Doug. I got up to use the bathroom and checked the time.

After what was probably about an hour, another staff member came with a gurney and told me they were taking me to the pre-op area. (I thought I was in the pre-op area, but I guess it was just the "pre" pre-op area.) I asked the tech if Doug could come, but the tech said he wasn't sure. We just decided to say good-bye at that point, but I later realized he could have come with me. We should have been a little more persistent. In the next area, the anesthesiologist, the surgeon, and the plastic surgeon all asked me where he was. At that point, though, I hoped my sweet boy had already had some breakfast and was headed back to the hotel room for a nap. I think they had given him a number to call or taken his number or set up some way of keeping track of my situation.

In the actual pre-op area, I met the anesthesiologist and the resident anesthesiologist. We talked about the fact that I would be intubated and that I would be under anesthesia for anywhere from 4-8 hours. He told me that they would watch me carefully and give me anti-nausea meds.

"I have struggled a lot with headaches post surgery," I told him when he asked if there was anything I was worried about.

"Ok, we can do our best to help with that," he said.

At this point, a nurse came and started the IV. I didn't get any meds yet, but I was ready to go IV wise.

Next came the plastic surgeon with a surgery resident and a plastics fellow. Dr. Le was bright, cheerful and struck me as a person who would be fun to have at a party. She had a pencil bag with her "tools"-a cloth tape measure (I think) and some surgical markers. She had me sit on the side of the gurney while she drew on my chest. Her two assistants, both men, were quiet and looked tired. They looked like babies to me, and I hoped they would be doing more watching than working.

I don't think I saw the general surgeon until two staff members came to roll me down a long hallway. To the left and right of the hallway were many, many doors. Each door was the entry to an operating room. I may be just imagining this, but I believe I was in O.R. #9. My name was written outside on a whiteboard along with the names of the anesthesiologist, the plastic surgeon, and the general surgeon. The procedures were also all written on the board. The general surgeon, Dr. Danford, was also there.

"Hello, Heidi," she said, "Good Morning! There are a lot of people behind those doors, and today, all of those people are here for you and we are going to take good care of you. We are all here for you." She repeated the "all here for you" part.

I felt calmer. I felt reassured. She has done this hundreds of times, I told myself-hundreds of times. She was confident and collected and today, I revered her. I was literally placing my life in her hands, and I appreciated the gravity of the situation. Inasmuch as I could, I understood the time and work and sacrifice it took for Dr. Danford to be standing there today in that OR ready to perform a bilateral mastectomy with a sentinel node biopsy in hopes of ridding my body of cancer. First she had completed four years of college, followed by four years of medical school. She then had to complete a five year general surgery residency followed by a breast fellowship (more training). I don't know how long the fellowship was or if she did additional years of training. Even after all that, it takes years, a huge part of a lifetime, before a surgeon hits his or her stride and achieves the skill level it takes to do what she was going to be doing for me that day.

I know, to a degree, what it takes to get to this place as a surgeon as Doug is an eye surgeon. It is years of nights and weekends of study and work and worry. He still agonizes over patients and is anxious the mornings he operates, not because he is not skilled, but because he is skilled and he still approaches each case with detail and care and precision. He appreciates the gravity of the situation each time he performs an eye surgery.

Once I was in the OR, I transferred from the gurney to the operating table. Dr. Danford introduced me to the folks in the room and someone got me positioned. They didn't start right away, but I knew they were about ready when Dr. Danford called a TIME OUT and asked me what I was having done. I realized that A TIME OUT is basically a situation where all the people in the operating room stop, pay attention, and listen to what procedure(s) is/are going to be done. I have had a number of surgeries done, but I have never been conscious during the TIME OUT. I had never seen the inside of the operating room. Someone asked me what procedure I was having done.

"I am going to have a bilateral mastectomy and have my expanders placed," I said.

Dr. Danford followed up, "We are also going to remove your port and do a sentinel lymph node biopsy. Is that correct, Heidi? Information on the sentinel lymph node biopsy is at the end of this post.

"Yes," I said, "I forgot about that."

With all that taken care of, the anesthesiologist stepped up next to me.

"Now I am ready to put you to sleep so we can start this for you, Heidi. I am going to inject some meds into your IV. I will be monitoring you very closely during the whole procedure and I will be checking on you when you come out of anesthesia. Do you have any questions?"

"No," I said, "I am just so relieved to be at this place. Let's get this party started."

And, within seconds, I was asleep. I had the easy part of the day. Doug had the hard part as did Jodi, my friend from Iowa, Grace, and my family. My mom and dad had taken the girls to Des Moines to meet my sister-in-law and her kids at the mall for the day. I am sure it was a crappy day for my mom and dad. I was grateful to my sister-in-law, Jody, for helping to keep everyone distracted. Later, Doug told me that Jodi and Grace had shown up before noon. The three of them had lunch and talked and passed the day. I think Doug got a nap in.

And I, well I was obviously under anesthesia and I don't remember anything. Dr. Danford performed the sentinel node biopsy and PRAISE THE LORD, there was no cancer in any of my lymph nodes. Her next and biggest job was the bilateral mastectomy. Before Dr. Le came in to start reconstruction, Dr. Danford had to make sure the margins were clear. Clear margins means no cancer cells are seen at the outer edge of the tissue that was removed. When the left breast was removed, it was immediately sent to the pathologists who were waiting and ready. Unfortunately, some cancer cells were still present, so Dr. Danford removed a little more tissue and sent the additional tissue back to pathology. Once she got the all clear, her part of the surgery was done, and she passed the baton to Dr. Le and her residents.

Of course, I knew none of this, but Doug was updated as the day went on. Dr. Danford called and told him that the lymph nodes were all clear. Then, Dr. Le started her part of the surgery.

I chose to have implant based reconstruction. Most of the volume of my new "foobs" would come from saline implants. I also chose to have these implants placed under the muscle instead of over the muscle. The permanent implants could not be placed immediately as the muscle needed to slowly stretch to accommodate them. So, a temporary tissue expander was placed and partially filled with saline. As I understand, most plastic surgeons detach the pectoralis major muscle from its lower starting point along the ribs and then place the implant under it. This type of surgery (versus over the muscle) can cause more pain as the implant is placed **under** the muscles. My tissue expanders had a magnetic port that the plastic surgery PA used post-surgery to do "fills" which were literally saline fills to make my "foobs" bigger.

What is a sentinel node biopsy for breast cancer?
Taken from Kaiser Permanente
A sentinel node biopsy is a type of procedure. It checks to see if breast cancer has spread to certain lymph nodes in your armpit. These are called sentinel lymph nodes. First the doctor injects a blue dye or a radioactive material into your breast. (In my case, I already had the radioactive marker and the dye placed the day before.) The dye flows through the lymph system to help the doctor find the correct lymph nodes. Then the doctor makes a small cut to remove your sentinel lymph nodes. Sometimes the doctor removes other lymph nodes too, if it looks like the cancer has spread. If the test shows that your cancer has spread to your lymph nodes, you and your doctor will discuss what you can do. Your doctor may remove more lymph nodes. Or you may decide to use chemotherapy or radiation. healthy.kaiserpermanente.org

DONE WITH SURGERY

JOURNAL ENTRY BY GRACE EDWARDS
DECEMBER 27, 2017

Hello,

Today Grace is writing a quick journal entry. I'm not the eloquent writer my momma is, but I'll try. Today Heidi went into the hospital at 5:45 a.m. Mom was in the pre-surgery unit until about 8:30 this morning. She went in, and doctors were able to successfully remove the small remainder of the tumor. The lymph nodes tested were negative, so that's a very good thing!! Now she is in a recovery room, and feeling pretty good. Hope to head home tomorrow. Looks good.

- Grace

Reflection

At about three in the afternoon, I was taken to the post-op area. I remember slowly coming to and my first question of the nurse was,

"Was the cancer in my lymph nodes?"

"No, it was not, and everything went really well," she said.

And that was enough.............That was all I needed to know. What do I remember about the rest of the day?

I remember talking to Doug and Grace and Jodi. I remember wanting to see my chest as soon as I was conscious. I remember that I had a catheter. I think I might have eaten that day, but I am not sure. I was in more pain that I imagined I would be in. The pain stopped me when I moved or tried to sit up. It took my breath away. It was like a wave that washed over me—it had a beginning and a middle and an end. When the pain passed with each movement, I took in a big breath of relief.

I stayed in the hospital room by myself that night which was perfectly fine. Doug and I are huge advocates of a good night's sleep, especially

Doug. I know that he NEEDS sleep, and I make sure he gets it. I am sure I was in and out of consciousness that night. I do remember that most of the nurses were men which surprised me a little. Why? I don't know? It shouldn't have. Sometimes you catch yourself in your own preconceived notions. My nurses were compassionate, but also let me know I was doing just fine and my pain was normal and appropriate.

Doug was back early in the morning, and I was up when he came through the door. It is cliche, but you really don't sleep much in the hospital at all. The nurses were in and out all night and we realized that I had not been receiving the muscle relaxant I was supposed to be getting. My chest muscles were angry and painful, and we started a muscle relaxant called Diazepam. (It started helping pretty quickly after I took the first dose.)

Doug wanted to arrive early so that he was present for rounds. For those who are not familiar with the term "rounds", here is an explanation.

Once a day, usually in the morning, a group of physicians, residents and other team members make "rounds" to check in on their patients who are hospitalized. As a patient, this is your opportunity to ask questions, discuss your progress, and determine when you can expect to be discharged. We had visits from the plastic surgery team, who decided to change the post-surgical bra to one size larger and from the general surgery team who checked on the drains and the incisions. Doug was most interested in speaking to the general surgery team.

"Do you know when the pathology report will be back?" he asked.

Dr. Danford responded, "Maybe later today, but it might be tomorrow. If it is later today, we will stop by and let you know. If not today, it will be tomorrow. We will plan on releasing you later today. We need to get the catheter removed and make sure Heidi can urinate on her own, help her shower, and make sure her pain is under control off the I.V. pain meds."

Doug was really fixated on the pathology report and, at the time, I was not at all fixated on that. I am not sure why I wasn't worried about the path report, because the results of the pathology report were very important in my long term prognosis. There is something called a residual cancer burden or RCB score that helps predict the likelihood of the cancer return-ing in TNBC and HER2 positive breast cancer patients. If there is no can-cer found at the time of surgery, the RCB score is 0 which is the optimal score. After 0, the next best score is 1. Very simply, a score of 2 means mod-erate risk and a score of 3 means a significant risk or cancer returning. The RCB score is calculated based on a number of factors according to Ingram.

> Seven fields are required to calculate the amount of remaining tumor burden — dimensions of residual disease in the tumor bed, percentages of overall cancer cellularity and in situ dis-ease, number of involved lymph nodes, and diameter of the largest metastasis — and patients are then classified as having minimal (RCB-I), moderate (RCB-II), or extensive (RCB-III) disease burden based on a continuous index.

"There's no special testing here, this is just organizing what we would otherwise report anyway in pathology, but doing it in a quantitative and standardized manner," explained Symmans, a pathologist at MD Anderson who holds a patent on the RCB tool (he said it would remain free).

This information is taken from "Residual Breast Cancer Tool Highly Prognostic After Neoadjuvant Tx— Tumor burden calculator predicted long-term outcomes in all breast cancer subtypes" by Ian Ingram.

I really did not know a ton about all of this, but all of this informa-tion had been on Doug's radar for a long time. He knew (I am glad that I did not) that my long-term prognosis depended on what the pathology showed. The whole day he was anxious, to the point where I was just,

"Doug, it is what it is—just calm down." His anxiety was adding to my anxiety.

Finally, a member of Dr. Danford's surgical team appeared with a copy of the pathology report. I could tell right away that Doug was not happy. He was agitated and was scrolling through his phone.

"I don't think this is right, Heid, they are saying you have an RCB of 2, but the calculator I have says you have an RCB of 1. I am going to ask Dr. Danford to stop by before she leaves for the day. It is just not right."

Honestly, I still didn't really get it. I was still in a post-surgical haze. I had gotten my catheter removed and every time I got up to use the bathroom I was in a lot of pain. Grace and Jodi were in the room with me; Grace was in the bed, and Jodi was in the chair.

My sweet, sweet friend, Kristin, and her husband, Mark, stopped in to see me later in the day. We got a picture together, and I showed Kristin and Mark my new foobs. Mark is a radiologist, so I figured the guy has seen a lot, and honestly, my boobs were not sexual anymore. I had bared them so many times that they were on the same sexuality level as a foot or a nose or a toe.

After they left, we started working towards the discharge process. Jodi helped me take a shower. I have talked to other patients who have had bilateral mastectomies and many were not able to shower for days. I was so happy to be able to shower. I am an "every day shower girl"-if not twice a day, so this made me feel human again. Jodi helped me in the shower. We have seen each other in the absolute best of times and the absolute worst of times. After her father died of cancer, I came to the hospital and sat with her. I saw his body after his soul had left this earth and moved to heaven, and I took her home from the hospital. We went to her house and started cleaning her room because her relatives would be coming. She was there with me after Grace was born and my father-in-law was dying and Doug had to go to Phoenix for a three-month-rotation and I had fallen apart with postpartum depression. We were college roommates. The joys and heartaches we have shared could be their own book, so suffice it to say that helping me shower did not phase either of us one bit.

After she left, one of the nurses came and showed Doug and I how to care for the two drains I had. He also gave us discharge instructions. Also, to Doug's relief, Dr. Danford stopped by and he was able to talk to her about the RCB calculator. She agreed with him that the calculations had been incorrect and that my RCB score was a 1. (The lower the number, the better the prognosis). It was close to five by the time I was ready for discharge, but we decided not to make the four hour drive back to Wausau. It was snowy and windy and dark.

Doug borrowed a wheelchair from the nurse's station and I held my bag on my lap. Grace carried a few other things and opened doors for us as we made our way back to our room at the Doubletree. We followed the same path we had taken just 36 hours before. I was tired and broken and weary, but still, my emotions were much calmer than when I had made the same journey a day and a half before.

POST SURGERY HAZE, DOUG'S POSSIBLE NEW CAREER AS A POST-MASTECTOMY NURSE, MY FABULOUS FOOBS, AND OUR FLOODED CABIN (IT'S JUST FUNNY AT THIS POINT!)

JOURNAL ENTRY BY HEIDI EDWARDS
DECEMBER 31, 2017

I am writing on Sunday with Property Brothers playing in the background (we sure could use those handsome brothers right now-more about this later). The pain post-surgery was worse than I had anticipated, largely because I had the expanders placed under the chest wall. The nurse I had Day One post-surgery said the use of expanders under the chest wall creates chest wall muscle spasms. It feels like there is a 24 inch wide rubber band squeezing around my chest making each breath I take painful. Moving in the wrong direction sends sharp shooting pains through my chest. Fortunately, I am taking a number of pain control meds in addition to an antibiotic and a stool softener. This combo of meds creates an odd sort of haze, and in all my dreams since surgery I always fight to wake up.

The nursing staff at the hospital were primarily men and they were wonderful. They were efficient and direct and kind and did not seem at all bothered by the fact that the placement of the drains (two) made it difficult to completely close my gown. My 44-year-old (not so beautiful) derriere was left exposed each time I made a trek to the bathroom. They (along with a wonderful nurse named Amie) emptied the drains with ease and reassured me that I was DOING GREAT. On Thursday afternoon, Amie taught Doug how to take care of the drains. I have a drain under each armpit that looks like a small grenade. When the suction on the drain starts to release and/or the drain is halfway full, the drain has to be emptied into a small cup, measured and recorded. When the output from a drain is 30 cc's or less for two consecutive days, the drain can be removed. It turns out Doug is pretty darn good with the drain care. He has been managing very well, and Grace is recording the output on her phone. I read on several online posts that this unique fluid/biohazard is amazing for plants, so we have been emptying the contents into a bonsai tree we were just gifted. We will keep everyone posted on the tree's progress. Doug also had to change all the dressings today and he did it like a skilled provider. I told him if ophthalmology falls through, he would make an AMAZING NURSE.

Moving on, I am shocked (in a good way) by the appearance of my new foobs (fake boobs). They are breathtaking. I am not saying this is a self-affirming way, but just because I never expected them to look so natural. Kudos to the plastic surgeon, Dr. Le, and her two kind fellows (fellows are doctors who are receiving additional training in plastic surgery after completing a general surgery residency). I will not have any feeling in these breasts, and I will have to consider nipple reconstruction options later, but so far, so good.

The last bit of INTERESTING NEWS came in the form of a phone call from our "Up North" neighbors yesterday afternoon. It seems that our furnace went out sometime in the last week and the EXTREME RECORD BREAKING COLD TEMPERATURES CAUSED one of the sprinkler system pipes to burst. Apparently, the damage is significant and impressive. (This is why we could use the Property Brothers.) It seems that 2017 had one last "surprise" for us. At this point, all we can do is laugh and say "What are the odds?" Honestly, it is really just funny. If I am OK, if my lymph nodes are clean, if my prognosis is positive, this is an annoyance. I do have to say it is an unlikely, crazy, shocking, unbelievable happening/event, but that's it.

Mom and Dad brought Ave and Lauren back today and they are here to propel us through the next couple of weeks. I have to go back to Mayo on Wednesday. Thank you to you kind folks who continue to bring us food. I plan to shut down the meal train at the end of January, but my-oh-my are we SO GRATEFUL FOR THE FOOD.

Ok, because my brain is SO SLUGGISH, it has taken me all day to write this. Posting now—with love, Heidi—Oh one last thing, Happy New Year! 🎈🥂

Reflection

As I write this, we are in the final stages of completing the cabin remodel—basically four years later. We are also in the midst of a global pandemic and a whole host of other devastating events in the US and around the world. Our cabin doesn't even deserve mention really, so forgive me. Last thing, the bonsai tree died! It did not like the post-mastectomy drainage.

RECOVERY, RECONSTRUCTION, RESTORATION

Journal Entry by Heidi Edwards
January 8, 2018

Today marks twelve days post-op, and I am feeling more like myself! I am not taking anything except Tylenol for pain. My main issue is that the muscles in my back are very, very tight and uncomfortable (perhaps because my whole posture is a bit different) and I can LITERALLY feel the expanders under my chest wall muscles. They really do feel like foreign bodies which is exactly what they are. Sleep is awkward and I alternate between the recliner in our bedroom and our bed. I sort of sleep in shifts—awake, asleep, awake, asleep. (That said, I know a lot of people are like that, so, in the words of my girls—whatevs). This morning, just when I had settled into a nice doze, Avery woke me up to ask me about riding lessons tonight. While I admit I was a little annoyed, it was really OK because I AM her Mom and she wants HER Mom to help her arrange her life, and I want to be her Mom, and I am glad that she comes to me. Her life has not and should not stop because my expanders make sleep elusive.

I saw a PA (Physician's Assistant) in the Plastic Surgery Department last Wednesday. She said everything looked good and removed the drain on the right side. Doug asked her if I could start exercising again, but she very gently told him I should wait for two weeks and then I could start going for walks. He feels like exercise is a big part of cancer prevention and recurrence, but vigorous exercise will have to wait. Moving around the house is fine, and I am doing a bit of housework here and there, but the truth is that I have been very BLESSED by the presence of my Mom and Dad who have taken over for me for a bit. Like my Grandma Marian was before her, my Mom is a gem in the kitchen and is much more careful with the laundry than I am, air-drying many items and ironing others that have never been ironed. She has mended a few things that I would have tossed.

Grace even offered her mending services to one of her friends. Grammy Judy is patient and kind with the girls. On Saturday she took Grace to a thrift shop called "Family Treasures" where she patiently waited for Grace to treasure hunt. Grace came home with a number of finds, including a pair of men's size medium Adidas pants that she drowns in and a pair of pink velour track shoes she describes as really "extra". She also found four barely worn really nice tops. She and my Mom got my Dad a red snowmobile jacket that he wasn't so sure about. He said he looks like Captain Kirk in it, and every time he puts it on he says, "Captain Kirk reporting for duty, sir." He tried to take it back today, but the Family Treasures lady stuck hard and fast to her no returns policy and Captain Kirk will stay on duty I guess. I scored an Eddie Bauer jacket from the trip as well.

Dad has been the main grocery shopper/errand runner/Louise walker. My dad also keeps me entertained with lots of very good stories about his own life experiences. For example, this morning he told me that when he first started teaching, he took his dress shirts and pants to a cleaner named Jim in southern Missouri. It cost him about twenty cents for a shirt and twenty cents for a pair of pants. He told me that he and Jim often flipped a coin for "double or nothing cleaning". If my Dad won the toss, Jim cleaned his shirts and pants for free. If Jim won, my Dad paid double. And so, I have had more one-on-one time with my parents than I have had in years and years and years. I am settling in and soaking that in and trying not to worry how long it takes to get back to baseline. My dad is OK as long as he has a job to do.

On Thursday, Doug and I will head back to Mayo to see the general surgeon's PA (physician's assistant), the plastic surgeon's PA, the oncologist, and a nurse (for an intro to survivorship visit). The plastic surgery PA will do a fill, using a port in each expander to inject more saline. (Essentially, my foobs will get a little bigger.) There is still a drain on the right side that she will remove as well. This fill process will continue periodically until my foobs are where I want them to be "size-wise". At an unknown time in the future, the expanders will come out and the permanent implants will go in. We will also talk to the oncologist (most important visit) to see what the next step will be treatment wise. I am not expecting to need radiation, but I might. There is also the possibility of six months of oral chemo. I am in the reconstruction phase now, not just breast-wise, but life-wise. I am, for now, recovering and resting, but I also am making plans for what I want to fill my time with once I am not in active treatment.

First on the list is cleaning up our flooded cabin. (A pipe burst the week of my surgery.) My sweet brother, a builder and roofer and construction expert, came up from Iowa last night to help assess the damage which is in his words "pretty bad". It's a bummer, but it could be fun to do a little bit of reconfiguring. Also, some of you have heard me tell you this a few times, so you are probably sick of it, but, after two-plus years of working on it, I GOT MY K-12 ESL TEACHING CERTIFICATION RIGHT BEFORE CHRISTMAS. I won't be teaching anytime soon, but who knows what the future holds.

This is the news from my "itty-bitty little corner" of the world. I know that so many of you are facing challenges and struggles, many equally or more taxing than mine. I hope for encouragement and peace for all of you, and strength in the year ahead.

And one more thing...........

PRAISE BE TO GOD FOR WALKING AHEAD OF ME AND BESIDE ME, AND FOR ANSWERING MY PRAYERS FOR A SUCCESSFUL SURGERY. THANK THE LORD THERE WAS NO LYMPH NODE INVOLVEMENT AND FOR GUARDING THE HEALTH OF ALL INVOLVED. LET GOD CONTINUE TO BE GLORIFIED IN THIS SITUATION.

Reflection

I am now in my third year of teaching at an elementary school in Wausau. I am the K-5 EL (English Language) teacher. I work Monday through Friday from 7:45-1:45 ish. Teaching during the pandemic has been its own story. Overall, it has been a really positive experience and it has given me purpose and meaning and a new set of social connections in students, families, and staff members.

TMI?

JOURNAL ENTRY BY HEIDI EDWARDS
JANUARY 15, 2018

I know this may be too much information for some of you, but I shared this story with the two Amy's (you know who you are) as a sort of a "litmus test". Their reaction gave me the courage to share it with a larger group of readers. In the midst of many heartbreaking situations, there is humor to be found and this narrative shares one of those humorous situations.

The night before my bilateral mastectomy, December 26th, Doug and I settled into our hotel room early. I was writing a bit and Doug, I think, was watching a little football (or something sports-related). Prior to my surgery, I had tried to prepare myself for the emotional impact of the mastectomy. I read what other women said and did, and a number mentioned photographing their breasts. Those who had done it were pleased and some who had not were regretful. Some even lived in hipper, artsier places where there were photographers who specialized in taking such photos. (Central Wisconsin would NOT be one of those places.)

Anyhoo....it was getting late, close to nine, and we were going to try to nod off early, and I got a little panicky. Certainly it was too late for anything professional. Grace is the best photographer in the family, and she wasn't with us. I tried a selfie, but it just wasn't working.

"Doug," I said, "do you think I will regret not taking some pictures of my breasts later on?"

"I don't know," he said, "do you want me to take a few?"

"I guess, maybe," I replied.

He remained in his horizontal position, and I "posed" (or something like that).

He snapped a few pictures, and when he was finished I looked at them.

"Doug, you took these from a terrible angle and they're awful! Can you at least sit up and try again?"

"Sure," he said, "but I don't really think it will make a difference."

He did sit up though and took a few more pictures. Still, though, they weren't attractive.

And then I realized the cold hard truth, the pictures were an accurate reflection of how my breasts really looked.

And as it turned out, the whole experience was helpful and I realized that maybe "getting new breasts" wasn't all bad. Sure, I would be losing sensation, but I would be getting smaller, perkier and maybe much nicer replacements.

We deleted the photos from our photo stream, but Doug messaged them to me and I decided that any time I feel a little mournful for my old breasts, I can refer back to the pictures and that will probably cheer me up.

It's been almost three weeks, and I'm really not sad about the mastectomy. Tomorrow I have another fill at Mayo (early in the morning), so my mom and I are heading there this afternoon. Today also happens to be my birthday, so we will celebrate with a fabulous meal and a nice night at my new favorite hotel in Rochester.

Last week on Thursday at a post-op Mayo visit, Doug and I had a chance to visit with the oncologist and she said I had a very good response to chemo and because of the mastectomy, I do not need any further treatment in terms of radiation or oral chemo. We are still not sure about whether or not to proceed with tamoxifen, but I will know that in the very near future.

So, for now, I am focused on the reconstruction process. Once the temporary expanders are full to the place I am comfortable with, I need to wait a minimum of three months before they can be exchanged with the permanent implants. I am hoping the exchange surgery can be done before summer so we can have an appointment free summer and I can be swimsuit ready! Ha! Ha!

Reflection

It has now been over two years since I completed the reconstruction process. I ended up not having the exchange surgery until August of 2018 (eight months post-mastectomy) because I needed to do about six months of oral chemotherapy. Then, I waited another year to have my nipple tattoos (August of 2019). I am basically happy with my new foobs. I wish I had gone a little bigger and my breasts are slightly asymmetrical. Dr. Le wanted to correct the asymmetry, but I am good for now. I am good for now. Plus, Doug said he is DONE with surgery. Asymmetry is sexy, right? Who wants perfect breasts?

WHERE DO I GO FROM HERE?

JOURNAL ENTRY BY HEIDI EDWARDS
JANUARY 29, 2018

Today is Monday, January 29th. For many weeks, Monday was my treatment day. When I started chemo, I didn't think too far into the future. I just kept my mind focused on getting through the treatments without interruption, staying well, taking care of the girls (and Doug), and living life as normally as possible. I finished chemo on November 27th. December came and I focused on making it through Grace's birthday, making it through Christmas, staying well, and preparing for surgery on December 27th. Since surgery, I have focused on recovery, the weekly trips back to Mayo, and living life as normally as possible.

And now, after this Thursday's trip to Mayo, I should be done with the plastic surgery appointments for a while. I think that this should be my final "foob" fill. Initially, I was told I needed to wait a minimum of three months before the exchange surgery where the tissue expanders will be removed and the permanent implants will be placed. (That has changed as I will be doing more chemotherapy. See paragraph below.)

From a cancer perspective, I will not be doing any hormone/endocrine therapy as some breast cancer survivors do since my triple negative status would make it ineffective/pointless. Initially, I thought I might end up taking Tamoxifen because there was a question about the receptor status, but the pathology report post-surgery stated that the remaining cancer was triple negative. I am also not doing any radiation because there was no lymph node involvement and because I opted to do a mastectomy instead of a lumpectomy. While my oncologist at Mayo did not recommend oral chemo, my oncologist at home (who I saw today) does recommend six months of an oral chemo drug called Xeloda. It is a sort of "insurance policy" on the chance that there are cancer cells remaining in my body. The hope is that the Xeloda would eliminate those cells. For the great majority of people, there are minimal side effects. While I was hoping to be "done", I am planning to go ahead with this medicine.

The way I see it, I can live with a few side effects, but I would be heartbroken if I had a recurrence and had not taken this drug. So, hello Xeloda! Hello to more trips to the Cancer Center! Hello to more blood work! Hello to more visits with my sweet oncologist! Hello to waiting longer for the implant exchange surgery! Oh well, this too shall pass........

This week marks the end of the meal train. I/we will be forever grateful for the meals that appeared at our house on Mondays, Wednesdays, and Fridays for over six months, each prepared by loving hands. I will be forever thankful for the dear friends who came to pick me up for treatment and who sat with me during treatment. I will be forever appreciative for each text and email that was sent to check-in and to encourage and for the cards and messages of hope that arrived in the mail. I will be forever touched by the gifts that wrapped me in love—blankets and books and bracelets and hats and gift cards and flowers and CHOCOLATE.

My mom and dad and brother and his family have been rockstars through all of this. Our family could not have lived as normal of a life as we did the past seven months without all the help of Lou and Judy.

The motto for CaringBridge (the site I used for these posts) is:

We believe that in times of need, the greatest source of hope and healing is the love of family and friends.

Dear friends and family,

In addition to the Lord, my greatest source of hope and healing has been, AND WILL CONTINUE TO BE, the love of family and friends.

With love for each and every one of you, Heidi

Reflection

Quite honestly, when Dr. Anand recommended Xeloda, I was heartbroken and angry. The next few posts reflect those emotions.

REQUEST FOR CONTINUED PRAYERS

Journal Entry by Heidi Edwards
February 7, 2018

Hello all-

I am in a hard place right now. I started the Xeloda last Saturday morning, and I was doing OK until yesterday morning. I take five pills in the morning and five pills in the evening. About an hour after taking the morning pills, I got very nauseous and threw up a number of times. It caught me off guard and I threw up in the twins' bathroom sink as I was collecting their laundry. I was able to talk to the pharmacist at the Cancer Center and Doug spoke with my oncologist. They both want me to try to stay on this dose and recommended I take an anti-nausea medicine, Zofran. I took it and it has helped. That said, I am discouraged. I am tired, but I still need to make it through these last six months. I am requesting prayers because PRAYER WORKS.

COURAGE DOESN'T ALWAYS ROAR

Journal Entry by Heidi Edwards
February 14, 2018

I nearly fell off the ledge this past week, but I think my feet are a bit more firmly planted now.

I started Xeloda on February 3rd. I will be completely transparent; I was not happy at all about it. I took the first five pills with anger, the next five with disappointment, and the next five with fear. Still, everything was relatively stable until Day Four when, a few hours after taking FIVE MORE STINKING PILLS, I started throwing up. I called the pharmacist at the Cancer Center, who advised me to take an anti-nausea pill, Zofran, with the next dose.

It did help, but the combo of Xeloda and Zofran, and my other supplements put me into a strange state. I felt less nauseous, but I developed new, frightening (frightening to me at least) symptoms—a foggy head with a sense of being off-balance, joint pain, and other issues. This upped my anxiety level to a ten out of ten. Were the symptoms medication related or had the cancer spread? Logically, I knew it was probably the meds, but a cancer diagnosis scares the crap out of a person and it is easy, in Doug's words, "to go down the rabbit hole". Once again, we put in a call to the Cancer Center.

At my oncologist's advice, I took a "two dose break" from Xeloda and felt SO MUCH BETTER. Monday, I was back at the Cancer Center where I visited with the very kind pharmacist and the oncologist who truly, truly dedicates most of his life to the practice of medicine. They talked me down from the ledge, and my oncologist reassured me that it was VERY UNLIKELY the cancer had spread and that the symptoms I was experiencing were quite likely med-related. He told me that the reason for the "two-dose break" was to see if my symptoms subsided, and the symptoms did. He/we decided to lower my 5000mg/day dose to 4000mg/day to see if that lessened the side effects.

So, I have taken four doses at the lower regimen. So far, so good! I think God played the most important role here. My mom and dad came last Thursday night, and we all prayed (all seven of us) for God's intervention in this situation. God is faithful.

Life is strange. I can parallel this current situation to a car trip. Maybe you started out in California, and you think the trip will be over when you get to Wisconsin. In fact, once you get to WI, the car is kind of trashed and your legs are tired. You are so glad to be done with eating on the road and sleeping in strange places. You are just relieved to be in WI. But then, you realize THE TRIP IS NOT OVER. You need to keep going; in fact, you need to keep going **all the way** to New York City. That is annoying and you whine and grump a bit, but eventually you just decide to clean out the car, gas it up, and GET MOVING. Maybe there are things you still need to see before your journey is over. Maybe there are lessons you still need to learn. Or maybe there is no discernable reason at all for why the trip isn't over. I finally got my mind wrapped around the fact that I still have a few miles to go. I am back in the driver's seat I guess, ready to keep driving.

A new friend in my life gave me a hand-lettered, framed piece of art at Christmas with the following words:

Courage doesn't always roar, sometimes it is the quiet voice at the end of the day that says I will try again tomorrow. (Thank you, CB, sister in the Lord.)

I realize that my challenge is not really that unique. Each of us have battles we are waging right now. Maybe some of you are like me and you are a little disheartened because you thought the battle was over, but it is not. And so, we stop and get our brave back (with the help of those we love and the Lord) and we try again tomorrow.

And maybe, just maybe, tomorrow is a little easier.

Reflection

A couple things come to mind as I re-read this post.

One of the best books I read during my cancer journey was *Find Your Brave*. It was gifted to me by my friend, Justine. I highly recommend this book along with my second favorite book, *There's No Place Like Hope*. *Find Your Brave* truly helped me "find my brave" during my cancer journey. I read it multiple times and have since gifted it to multiple people.

Finding out that I had to take the Xeloda, starting it, and feeling so strange at the outset was a very low point in my cancer journey. I was just mentally feeling like I was done post-surgery, and I was very discouraged that I wasn't. Around the same time that I started the Xeloda, I also started another medication called tetrathiomolybdate (a sort of experimental med for TNBC). I don't know if it was the Xeloda or the combination of the two, but the six months that I took the Xeloda were trying for me.

I did nearly have a breakdown during the first Xeloda cycle. One night, during the first Xeloda cycle (a cycle was two weeks on the drugs and one week off), Doug and I pulled into the garage at the same time. We both got out of our cars at about the same time and I told him I couldn't do it (the Xeloda) and I was falling apart. I don't remember exactly what he said to me, but it was something like, "You cannot fall apart, do you understand, you cannot fall apart. I am only keeping it together because you are keeping it together. If you fall apart, I will fall apart." Then he walked out of the garage. I stood there for a while, and I literally walked back in the house having decided I would keep it together.

Probably right after the garage incident, Doug, unbeknownst to me, called my Mom and Dad and asked them if they could come up for a while. They did, and they got us through another rough patch. I remember that while they were here, we went and looked at campers at a place called King's Campers. I walked through the showroom kind of numbly, sitting in different campers that all had a new camper smell. We talked to a salesperson that was hopeful for his first February sale. I knew there was a one in a million chance my parents would buy a camper from this nice Northwoods guy. They were WAY too practical for that kind of monkey business. (Just having fun here-I think campers are the bomb.com, but my parents are WAY too practical for one.) Still, I knew they were just trying to get me out of the house and distract me; I knew that and they knew that and it worked-as much as it could. The weight of everything was still with me, but I knew what my wise parents were trying to teach me. They were teaching me that the weight was not so heavy that it stopped me. Even though I might be moving a little bit slower, I could still move. The morale of the story:

Parents never stop parenting, even when their daughter is 45. (I am 48 at the time of writing this reflection.)

KIND OF DEEP HERE

JOURNAL ENTRY BY HEIDI EDWARDS
MARCH 5, 2018

An old and precious friend, Michelle, recently shared a podcast with me from a woman named Kate Bowler. Kate is a professor of religion at Duke Divinity School. At age 35, Kate was diagnosed with stage 4 colon cancer. This prompted her to write a book called *"Everything Happens for a Reason: And Other Lies I've Loved."* In the book, she realizes that she unconsciously subscribed to the belief that if she just "believed" enough and "worked hard", she could somehow control her destiny. She says, and I am paraphrasing here,

"What did I expect from life? I expected things to really just work out. Then, after my diagnosis, I realized that maybe life is just vine to vine—hanging on to dear life."

She also discusses how her faith has been affected by her diagnosis. Kate is an expert in the "prosperity gospel", a belief that financial and blessings are the will of God for believers. In other words, if you have faith in God, he will deliver health and wealth to you. Kate did not necessarily subscribe to this theology, but she was well-versed in it. Her diagnosis forced her to re-examine her beliefs.

To a large degree, I totally understand where she is coming from. I do not subscribe to the "prosperity gospel" because I understand that sometimes/oftentimes God's will is not my will. My will is to live a long life, to watch my girls grow up, to retire with Doug and maybe spend winters in Florida or Arizona or someplace warm. I want to teach more ESL, travel and see the world. I believe in prayer and I believe that God hears prayer. I hope, in regards to cancer, that my will is his will. This topic could be the subject of an entire book, and I am not even touching it here. For those reading this, I recognize the inadequacy of this post in relation to faith.

Of course, I do know that all of our lives are uncertain. None of us know what the future holds, but before my diagnosis I did not question my future nearly as much. Like Kate, I took much more for granted. Like Kate, I wish that I could go back to that place (before cancer) because it was more peaceful.

I can't though. And I have found a clarity that I did not have before. Grace told me that she has not seen Doug and I argue since July; she is right, we haven't. I am taking the time to just sit with the girls in whatever they are doing and not hurry or think about what I need to get done. I am more sympathetic and empathetic to the struggles that people are enduring. I am grateful for each day that I feel good and for each day that I can do what I want to do.

I am also blessed right now because I am peaceful and OK emotionally. Physically, God has answered my prayers and I am doing well with the Xeloda. I will finish my second of eight rounds on Friday and will be 25% done. Yeah!!

Reflection

I still have not read Kate's book, but I am putting that on my "to do" list. I just googled her and it looks like she is still doing well, and I am very grateful for that. On her web page, she mentions that she hopes her cancer will move (in the future) from being life threatening to being almost like a chronic illness. I pray that science is moving towards a reality like that. Also, as time has passed and now I am already four years post-diagnosis, I realize that I am not as present as I was immediately post-cancer. It is good for me to re-read this post and remind myself to slow down, especially with my daughters. I hope that I am still empathetic and sympathetic to the struggles and pain of others. I am deeply grateful for my health. I keep a little prayer/gratitude journal and I thank God for my health EVERY day, a practice I plan to continue for life.

WISDOM FROM THE PATIO DOOR

Journal Entry by Heidi Edwards
March 19, 2018

Since I was diagnosed with cancer, I am more attentive to social media posts, TV shows, news articles, etc. about stories related to cancer, especially personal stories. Of course not all patients share this sentiment, but there are definitely some who say that their life is richer/better/more meaningful post-diagnosis.

Hmmm.........

I tend to be a more middle-of-road girl. In lots of ways, this whole experience SUCKS. I have spent WAY TOO MUCH time in doctors' offices and waiting rooms this past year. I have lost my hair and my breasts. I have been nauseous and depressed and scared.

But.........

Life HAS BECOME more in focus, sharper and clearer. One day (in February) I was listening to a podcast while cleaning off the kitchen desk. The speaker was sharing his own experiences in caring for his father with Alzheimer's. He stated that his experiences changed the lens he looked at his life through. He stated that the struggle of caring for his dad made him ask some important questions.

1. What am I doing? (in life)
2. Where am I going? (in life)
3. Who do I want to be? (in life)

The journey he was taking with his dad brought these questions to light. I really like them. When I heard this part of the podcast, I paused, listened again, and then grabbed a dry erase marker and wrote them on my patio door. They have been there for at least a month. I windex (Windex would love that I have made a verb out of their product) the door at least once a week, but the words stay. And, I plan to rewrite them when the words start to fade, just as I plan to "rewrite" parts of my life if I don't like the answers to the questions. The questions cancer makes you ask do bring focus and clarity to one's life.

Another piece of wisdom from the speaker was this:

Healing is receiving love.

I had to repeat this mantra over and over to let its power sink in. Healing IS receiving love. We can be healed ourselves and we can help heal others.

Ok, that's my teeny bit of wisdom for the day.

I am doing well. I started my third 14-day cycle of Xeloda on Friday. After tonight's dose I will have four days under my belt. That is a happy thing. I have a nice head of hair now, and I don't think I will dye my hair again. The Edwards girls are running again. Grace's track season started on March 5th and she had her first indoor meet on Saturday. She is pretty serious about track. The littles start today. Ave wasn't too sure about it, but I assured her "she was going to love it!" Lauren is a go for any activity where she can get a t-shirt or sweatshirt with the team logo. Doug is just keeping on keeping on and providing a strong and stable presence for all the crazy women in his life, and that is no small task.

Reflection

None of the Edwards girls are running track anymore. Grace's freshman year, while very successful, was her one and only year of high school track and field. I think track and field is a pretty exciting sport, but the meets are very long. Lauren and Avery ran as 7th graders, and there was not an 8th grade season due to COVID. Neither of them ran as 9th graders. Lauren talks about running this year. We will see.

I have still not dyed my hair again despite going back and forth about whether to trade in the gray for my dark brown pre-cancer color. In March of 2021, when our family traveled to Arizona for spring break, Doug and I found ourselves waiting in the rental car line while the girls parked themselves in another area of the rental area. The associate greeted us with,

"You guys must have the grandkids along if you are renting a minivan." I often get asked if I want the senior discount at Trig's and Lamb's Fresh Market (both local supermarkets) while doing my grocery shopping. These moments make me consider going back to the beauty aisle, buying a box of hair dye, and doing it myself, but I have yet to do so. We will see. Pictures of my mom and I are funny as I have gray hair and she does not.

I do not have any of these questions on my patio door anymore, but re-reading this post today makes me realize I should probably get out my whiteboard marker and write them again. COVID has created some interesting scenarios for a lot of people, including our family. These questions are just as relevant as ever-maybe even more so.

WE SHOULD LIVE ON A FARM/MY POOR FEET

Journal Entry by Heidi Edwards
April 9, 2018

Today is April 9th, and THERE IS STILL SNOW ON THE GROUND—LOTS OF IT!

By this time last year, spring had sprung. In fact, early in the morning of April 10th of 2017, we had a little tornado in our neighborhood. We were the last house the tornado hit, taking out most of the small forest in our backyard and all the trees in our front yard. The F-1 category tornado (official categorization by the National Weather Service) also blew in one of our garage doors, caused extensive damage to our roof, deck, and screened in porch, and demolished our trampoline. The loss of all the trees created a whole new view. Little did we know it would be a sign of more changes in our life and the necessity of seeing life from a different perspective.

Back to the topic of spring.............

For Grace, spring has meant the start of the high school track season. Track started March 5th and the indoor track season will finish up this week. Hopefully the snow will be gone soon so the team can practice outside and start the outdoor season. She has been running the 800 and the mile. Go West Track!

For the littles, spring has been an effort to acquire new animals. In Lauren's case, she really, really wants to be able to raise chickens in our backyard. For some time, there was talk about our township changing the regulations to allow for this. Because we weren't sure what the rules were, Lauren (on her own) found the correct town official to email. Using my email account and posing as me, she has been emailing back and forth with this patient man. She was devastated to learn that chickens ARE NOT ALLOWED. However, she replied back to this denial wondering if and when the law might change asking if there is "anything we could still do to get chickens". I am sure this man thinks I am crazy.

Avery is on a quest for bee hives and a "pig". Last night, before bed, she told me she already has a name picked out for the pig-Hamlet or Bacon. She told me that if the town doesn't allow pigs, the pig can live inside. Apparently, they are smarter than dogs and much easier to potty train. She strengthened her case by telling me the litter box could be in her room, the pig could sleep at the end of her bed, and she would get up with it at night. None of these promises strengthened her case. We ended our bedtime conversation by deciding that:

1. We should have lived on a farm.
2.   I would not officially say no to the pig request, but just "think about it".

Moving on.....................

From a cancer perspective, I am living my "short-term" new normal. I am on Xeloda cycle 4 of 8 right now. It is going just fine. I am not having nausea, just fatigue and muscle aches. The biggest complaint, however, is the hand (or in my case) foot issues. This medicine dilates the capillaries in the hands and feet. Heat, friction, and pressure can make the capillaries burst and cause lots of foot (or hand) pain and blisters. During spring break, we went to Florida. On our second day, I went for a 1.5 mile walk with Doug on the beach without shoes. By about halfway through, my feet started really hurting. An hour later, I had big blood blisters on both feet. So, I did not walk too much the rest of the week. I spent a lot of time sitting and icing my feet by filling plastic grocery bags full of ice.

I do have one funny story about this though.

G has turned into a serious thrifter, and we visited a few thrift stores in Florida. At one thrift store, while hobbling around, I found a pair of huge, white orthopedic shoes for only three dollars. I was hopeful that these pretty darn ugly shoes might provide some relief, and I bought them (much to the girls' dismay). They were missing the inserts, though, so Doug stopped at Walgreens and bought me some gel inserts. I carefully cut them down to size, and tried them on. It wasn't pain-free walking, but the new shoes weren't too bad. I wore them around for a few hours before the sole started falling off and leaving a trail of a white, powdery substance almost like sand. Sadly, I had to throw away my "find" when the sole on the left foot actually fell off. :(

Life always has some laughs if you look hard enough. I am happy to report that my feet are improving and I am very, very careful with them right now. I always wear shoes, moisturize a lot and keep my tootsies out of any hot water.

Reflection

We really should have lived on a farm because now we are in the horse business in a serious way. In the fall of 2019, we bought our first horse, Rusty. By we I mean Doug and I. We bought the horse, but Avery rides, trains and cares for him. In the summer of 2020, Avery had the chance to take a trip to South Dakota with another family who is heavily involved with horses. Their daughter told Avery about a program through the American Quarter Horse Association (AQHA) called the Youth Development Program that she had participated in. Essentially, adult members of the AQHA donate weanlings to youth members who are selected through an application process. In 2020, about 100 applicants applied and about 40 youth received a weanling. Avery was one of the lucky applicants who was chosen and Doug, Lauren, Avery and Avery's friend traveled to South Dakota at the end of October in 2020 to pick up RWS Silver Luxury a.k.a. Lux (names chosen by Avery) from the Raymond Sutton Ranch in Gettysburg, South Dakota. He was still nursing when they picked him up and just over three months old. Doug and I were a little leery about all of this, but agreed to allow Avery to participate under the condition that she would assume financial responsibility for baby Lux, a task she has taken on admirably. She works at the barn where her boys live two nights a week and is able to make enough money to pay for Lux's board, feed, ferrier, and vet bills. She is also currently working with a third horse, Ivy, that just turned three.

She is heavily involved with horses which means Doug and I are heavily involved with horses. Besides school and home, the barn is where Avery (and I) are most frequently.

Update since the reflection-things in the horse world are always changing

Avery sold Rusty and bought another horse, Cutie Pie, which she has re-named Lola. If all this is confusing to you, the reader, I apologize. I will just say my 15-year-old negotiated the sale of Rusty and purchase of Cutie Pie a.k.a. Lola all by herself. This mama is amazed by her business sense and initiative. (She did need money from us, though!)

Lauren still wants chickens, but so far no go. Maybe life will offer her the chance to live on a farm and own some chickens. I am hopeful for her. Avery's ag class this spring was looking for adoptive homes for the chickens they hatched, but I held firm on my refusal.

Grace is still a serious thrifter and has a frequent shopper card at Goodwill. She and her sisters (mostly Lauren because Ave is usually at the barn) like to hit Goodwill, Family Treasures, St. Vincent de Paul, Nice as New and a few others regularly. Grace has an affinity for Harley Davidson apparel and personalized work attire-someone else's. She is currently into oversized items and with a pair of simple sewing scissors she transforms oversized "blah" into "hip and trendy". She is not afraid to cut and use the sewing machine Papa Lou got for us at a garage sale to create new and interesting combinations. The rest of us aren't sure if her creations will always hold together, but Grace is undeterred. Grace recently started college at UW-Madison, and I am sure that she will quickly gain familiarity with the thrift store scene in Madison.

KIDS AND CANCER

Journal Entry by Heidi Edwards
April 30, 2018

When I was first diagnosed, my primary concern (after myself), was the girls. Immediately, I worried about dying and leaving them without a Mom. That concern is still there, but I feel much more optimistic about my long-term survival.

They found out about the cancer diagnosis at the same moment I did, and we all sat on our green cabin sofa and cried together. I am sure that memory will be etched in their brains forever. I think the whole experience has been more difficult for Grace than the twins because she "gets" it and understands the seriousness of the situation. Now that we are basically ten months into dealing with cancer, I think I have learned a bit about helping kids navigate this tender time in a family.

1. You have to be honest with them. We were honest from "Day One" and didn't sugarcoat the situation. We told them it was serious, but that my chances looked pretty good. We never promised anything. We shared what was happening each step of the way.

2. You have to get them involved in the process. We all went together as a family when I got my head shaved, and we all went wig shopping. Lauren and Avery went with me to a make-up session for cancer patients which reminded me of a TV sitcom and pretty much cracked us up. We all did the Susan G. Komen together and Grace was there when I spoke at our local Volley for the Cure. She also really wanted to be with Doug when I had my bilateral mastectomy. I had thought it would be better for her to be with my Mom and Dad, but

she just needed to be there and see what was happening as it happened.

3. In as much as humanly possible, you have to still be THE MOM. Sometimes others want to protect you from fighting kids and parental stress, but your kids still need to know that you are in control. They need the routine of YOU tucking them in and helping them pack for their three days at the school forest or the cross-country meet. They need to know that they can still share their problems with you, and that you aren't too fragile for that.

4. You have to let them know what they can do to help the family. One of the best things we did as a family was walk. I told them that exercise would really help me, and that their support in walking with me was HUGE. So we walked and we talked and we laughed. Sometimes, we had some complaining, but we still always finished our walks.

5. You have to keep the routine because kids need routine (and so do adults). Many folks, especially my Mom and Dad, helped with keeping our normal routine.

6. You have to keep others in the loop. At the beginning of the year, I let the girls' guidance counselors know what was happening in our family. Grace's guidance counselor called her down to the office and said (according to Grace), "I understand your Mother is not well." To which Grace responded, "She has cancer." The kind woman asked, "Would you like to talk about it?" To which G responded, "Nope." And the wise woman sent her back to class, but at least Grace knew that the support was there if she needed it. I asked the counselors and teachers to let me know if anything came up with behavior/grades/friendships that they were privy to.

7. You have to let them know that other kids (especially middle and high-school kids) might not know how to react and

might not be able to give them the support they might want. Interestingly, it seemed like Lauren and Avery's friends found it easier to ask them about the cancer than G's friends. I surmise that older kids worry more about saying the wrong thing.

8. You have to remember that even though you might be in the fight of your life, your kids are still kids. They will still fight over who gets to wear what or who folded more of the clothes in the ONE load you asked them to fold. They will still forget their instruments at home or need you to bring their track bag to school. They will still cry over a friendship struggle or whack each other over the last piece of gum.

9. Sometimes, you have to pull in a little and be with each other and love on each other.

Ok, here's my disclaimer..........

I hope I don't come off as sounding like I know it all, because that is FAR FROM THE TRUTH. I just wanted to get these thoughts down because I don't want to forget them.

Disclaimer #2

I have said this before, but I know that our struggle is just one struggle among millions of struggles. I know that so many are hurting and in pain, and that I am not unique.

OK—just a quick update on my progress.

I am halfway through the Xeloda! I started my fifth of eight cycles last Thursday night. I am moving along and swallowing four red pills in the morning and four red pills in the evening. My feet have healed from a nasty hand/foot syndrome outbreak, and my spirits are good. For those of you living in Wisconsin, you know that we had an amazingly long winter with record-breaking amounts of snow. Seeing the grass and feeling the sun is a gift from God and a real boost to one's morale.

Blessings-Heidi

Reflection

I recently asked the girls what they remember about my cancer journey and they had little to say. All of them remember the diagnosis and the surgery and Grandma and Papa coming a lot. They didn't want to talk about it much, though. Grace said, "That was a hard time in my life and I don't want to talk about it." I hope we did OK with all things related to kids and cancer. I have been following the journey of a young dad named Brandon Janous. He lost his wife, Rachel Janous, to triple negative breast cancer in early 2020. He chronicled this loss on his Facebook and Instagram pages and he is now speaking so eloquently about parenting after the loss of his wife. I know that could have been me. I know that. I don't know why God gave me the gift of time he has given me. It is not because I am more worthy or more needed. I probably won't know the answer to my question this side of heaven.

MAY NEWS

JOURNAL ENTRY BY HEIDI EDWARDS
MAY 30, 2018

It has been almost a month since my last post.

I guess it means that the time I spend thinking about breast cancer lessens each week. Imagine a pie chart. For about nine months of the last year, if I had made a pie chart of what was commanding my attention, cancer would have taken up at least half the circle. Now, it seems like cancer would only take up about 20-25% of the circle. That's a good thing. It hasn't been a deliberate change, but one I just noticed in the past week.

I still have blood work and oncology visits every three weeks. I still take about 30 pills a day. Eight of those are the oral chemo, but the rest are vitamins and supplements and a few prescription meds. Tomorrow I will finish cycle six of eight of the Xeloda (oral chemo). If all goes as planned, I will be done in mid-July. The side effects are manageable, the worst being my feet. They don't like pressure or heat and are super sensitive, but it's fine, though, really fine.

The past month I have been able to work outside pulling weeds (with a mask) and planting a little garden. I have switched out all the winter gear for summer gear. I have been able to attend lots of track meets. I have LOVED celebrating the graduations of lots of special folks. The Memorial Day weekend was filled with some wonderful times with friends, and I am gearing up for summer and for having the girls HOME.

Just a while after I was diagnosed, I talked to a woman in Seattle who had just finished up with treatment. She said, "I know it is hard to believe, but a year from now, you will find yourself sitting on a beach (or somewhere special) and you will be done. It won't be nearly as hard as it is now."

I didn't really believe her then, but I do now.

I know I am not out of the woods yet. My oncologist said if I am still cancer free in three years, we can bury the hatchet. I said, "I don't know if I will ever be able to 'bury the hatchet'".

He responded, "Well, if you don't, I will make you."

I love that guy, and I am starting to believe it all might just be OK.

Reflection

Today's date is May 20th, 2021. My 45-year-old self would not/could not have imagined or predicted what the next three years would bring. What we as a world have experienced since early 2020 is something we could have never imagined or predicted, kind of like cancer. I have fared very well during the pandemic, mostly because I did not lose anyone close to me. A second, but equal factor, was the fact that I had recently been through a harrowing experience. I am feeling much better about my prognosis and I probably only think about cancer for five minutes a day now, but I haven't buried the hatchet quite yet. Maybe in one more year. Grace, just today, had her last day of high school at West. This week, on May 18th, Doug and I celebrated 25 years of marriage.

Post-Script:

I am editing this on October 9th 2021, and COVID is still a very real and present part of the landscape.

JUNE NEWS

JOURNAL ENTRY BY HEIDI EDWARDS
JUNE 27, 2018

It's summer!

Since last summer SUCKED (I don't really like that word, but it seems appropriate here), I am bound and determined to just soak up every bit of pleasure I can from summer this year. So far, so good............

The girls finished up school on June 7th. On Monday, June 11th, we took off for Iowa. Our first stop was Waverly, Iowa. After a good night's sleep at a local hotel, we took a short walk to Wartburg College, the college where Doug and I attended. Grace is only going to be a tenth grader, but since we were in the area, we did a tour with my college roomie and forever friend, Jodi, and her daughter who will be a senior next year. We had a great time; the girls' favorite attraction at Wartburg was an enclosed area where six tortoises spend half the year. We were able to feed them and Grace said the tortoises were reason enough to go to Wartburg.

On Wednesday the 13th, we drove to Cedar Rapids, Iowa where we met my sister-in-law, Jody, and my two nieces and my nephew. We were able to have dinner with some MORE family in Cedar Rapids and in the morning, the two moms and six kiddos got on a flight to Fort Myers Beach where we had a cousin/sis-in-law week. We didn't have any big plans—just the pool, the beach, ice cream, and a little bit of shopping. The cousins fell into an easy rhythm with each other and it didn't seem like five months had passed since they saw each other last. I love my sis-in-law, Jody, so I had a blast, too.

A week later (Wednesday the 20th) we were back at home. The next day (Thursday the 21st) we were able to enjoy a noon lunch downtown—dining on cuisine from local food trucks. Friday night (the 22nd) we had some new friends over for dinner and on Saturday (the 23rd) some old friends invited us for a day at their lake house.

I love it all..............every day, every experience, and every person. I am grateful in a way that I wasn't last year. I was diagnosed on July 5, 2017, so next week I will be ONE YEAR FROM DIAGNOSIS. Last year at this time it was so hard to know what the year ahead would be like.

In terms of the cancer journey, I am starting my last cycle of oral chemo TOMORROW. I should be done on July 11th. I have already scheduled my exchange surgery for August 24th at Mayo. At this time, the temporary tissue expanders will be exchanged for permanent silicone implants. Yesterday, I was walking with my friend at a local park. I was explaining the exchange process to her. As I was explaining this, I cupped my foobs with my hands and said, "These girls are about to be upgraded." An older gentleman standing nearby saw me (and maybe heard as well). He looked at me and gave me a big wave and a smile. OH BOY!!! I decided it was time to hop in the car and head off.

Once I finish the oral chemo, I will be monitored every three months (I think). Triple negative BC tends to recur, if it is going to recur, in the first three years. The prayer of my heart is, of course, complete healing, and a life free of cancer.

For any of my local friends, the Susan G. Komen for North-Central WI will be on August 12th—starting on the 400 block. I started a team called Heidi's Heroes. We would love to have a whole crew of friends running and/or walking with us.

Reflection

I realize, as I read this post, how lucky I was when I was going through all of this to have such strong family support and also financial resources. It was huge. I know that this is not everyone's situation, and in writing this I recognize (of course) that my experience is not everyone's experience. But still, women going through a cancer journey share many common experiences. I hope that any woman or man going through cancer will find some hope by reading my narrative.

I DIDN'T KNOW IF I WOULD GET HERE, BUT I DID!

JOURNAL ENTRY BY HEIDI EDWARDS
JULY 11, 2018

I was diagnosed on July 5, 2017, at about 9:00 a.m. We were up North for the holiday weekend when the pathologist called Doug and our whole lives changed in a moment.

After the call, I stood in the kitchen wearing an old t-shirt and Doug's jacket (that was much too big for me) and just sobbed.

We didn't really know at that point what the diagnosis meant. We didn't know if I would be alive in a year or not.

Fortunately, within a few weeks, we were much more optimistic about the outcome, and felt very hopeful. Still, it felt like we were going on a journey without a map or a well-packed suitcase.

As I mentioned previously, I remember talking to another breast cancer survivor a few months after diagnosis and she said,

"I know it is hard to believe, but a year from now you will be sitting on a beach somewhere or at a restaurant with friends or just at home, and you will be OK."

I don't know if I believed her or not, but I do REMEMBER ALMOST WORD FOR WORD what she said.

And she was right...................IT'S JULY 11TH today and I am OK.

On July 5th this year, Doug, Grace, and I spoke just for a moment about the fact that it had been a year since that awful morning, and then we just went about our day. I was not quite ready for celebrating yet, but I knew DARN WELL what day it was.

Today, July 11th, seems more celebratory to me because tonight I will take my last dose of Xeloda! It has been 23 weeks since I started. When I started on them, I honestly didn't know if I would be able to complete the 8 dose cycle (2 weeks on, 1 week off, 8 pills/day during the on weeks).

But, I did, and it was the love of family and friends and the GRACE of God that sustained me. I can do all things through HIM who strengthens me. Phillipians 4:13

I am still trying to make sense of what I am supposed to do with this experience. I still feel like I am in a haze sometimes, but I am starting to put my life back together again. I am planning to teach again at the local university in the fall. I want to be a youth group leader at church as well. Lauren and Ave are starting to forget about the cancer a bit and the word cancer isn't spoken in our house every day. I know, though, that I have to do something meaningful with this experience. In addition to getting back to "my life", I have to find a way to advocate for others facing cancer.

I pray that the cancer does not recur and I continue to ask for prayers on my behalf regarding this. I know it is possible, and it is frightening. Every time I have an ache or pain, my immediate thought is—cancer. I think that fear will be present for a long time.

Last Friday, July 6th, Doug and I went to Mayo to meet with the plastic surgeon. On August 24th, my tissue expanders will be removed and the permanent implants will be placed. At the appointment, I was able to choose the implants I wanted. I went with the "not too hard, not too soft, right in the middle" implants. This procedure should not require an overnight hospital stay. Instead, I will have surgery early and be released late in the day. The surgeon did ask that I spend one night post-surgery in Rochester.

It seems that the finish line is finally in sight. It has been a long race. I didn't do it alone though. There was always someone (or lots of someones) right by my side.

Reflection

That Xeloda was hard. I hated it. It made me feel really weird and made me really tender towards people who are on maintenance chemotherapy. I know that there are many, many cancer patients who will never be "cured". Instead, cancer is a chronic condition that is managed as much as possible and for as long as possible. Finishing the Xeloda was a huge milestone for me. Coincidentally, I was going out for dinner with two of my friends the night of my last dose. I waited until I got home to take the last four pills with Grace and Doug in the kitchen with me, though. I wanted to share that moment with them and celebrate with them.

THE STATUTE OF LIMITATIONS ON CANCER/
COME AND CELEBRATE WITH US!

Journal Entry by Heidi Edwards
August 8, 2018

Last week we spent most of the week at the Wisconsin Valley Fair. Avery (well really, Doug and I) are half-leasing a beautiful six-year-old Gypsy horse named Bailey. The big reason we have been leasing Bailey was so Avery could take her to the fair. My knowledge of horses and what you do with horses at the fair was quite limited until last week. Now I understand A LOT more about what it means to "take a horse to the fair". It really is a week commitment with five of the days being about 15 hour days. Avery and I were at the fair by about 7 a.m. in the morning and Doug and Avery didn't leave until between nine and ten. Bailey needed to be fed and watered often, and horses poop much more than I could have ever imagined. They basically (it seems to me) poop as much as they eat. Each day of the fair brings a different style of competition—English, Western, Gymkhana, Trail. Also, each style necessitates unique apparel and unique types of saddles, etc. Avery really enjoyed the experience; Doug and I found it very interesting. The extensive time at the fair allowed for quite a bit of chatting with other parents. One day, while standing by the arena, another Mom asked me how I was doing. I responded by telling her that I had finished my oral chemo about three weeks ago, but that I was still getting my life back together. I mentioned that to others it was kind of over, but it wasn't really over for me. She shared the fact that her nuclear family had suffered with the deaths of a number of grandparents a few years ago. She said, "Personally, I needed to grieve for a long time, but after a while, people got a bit tired of hearing about it. I had reached my statute of limitations on grieving." Her comment kind of resonated with me. At a certain point, there is a statute of limitations on cancer, too. I have definitely reached it with the kids. MAMA IS BACK IN THE HOUSE. That said, a statute of limitations isn't really a bad thing for a number of reasons. First of all, there are literally millions of people who are facing situations much worse than breast cancer, and I am not the only one to go through some suffering. Secondly, sometimes you need a little push to get back in the game. I don't think it would be good to keep sitting in that place called "being a cancer patient". Right now, I am well. Right now, I am not sick. I have a good chance of never having to deal with a recurrence, so I am looking forward. That is the only place I can look.

I am looking forward to the Susan G. Komen Race for the Cure on Sunday.

We were hoping to do a little pre-/post-race party, but the timing just didn't work out. So, we are looking forward to hosting an ice-cream social on Sunday, August 19th from 5-8 p.m. at our house. This is a chance to celebrate the end of a long journey and a chance for me to get a good-luck hug before my August 24th surgery. :) We hope you can come celebrate with us!! Please shoot me a text or an email and let me know if you plan to attend, along with a head count. Please bring lawn chairs, kiddos, dogs, etc.

I would like to mention that Louise and Lauren made quite a pair at the Wisconsin Valley Fair's Dog Show! Louise was a blue (and red) ribbon dog!

Reflection

The implant exchange was not a big deal at all. I waited another year (2019) before getting nipple tattoos in Mankato, MN. Once I had committed to the idea of a bilateral mastectomy with reconstruction, I started following a guy named Vinnie Myers. Vinnie is located in Baltimore and has a team of tattoo artists who specialize in nipple and areola tattoos post-mastectomy. I had planned on traveling to Baltimore until I discovered that one of the artists, Trent Wyczawski, who had previously worked for Vinnie, had moved to Mankato, MN, a much closer option for me. I pulled this right from the Mecca Tattoo website:

"Trent Wyczawski has been tattooing for the past 15 years in Baltimore, MD. In addition to traditional tattooing, for the past 5 years he has specialized in medical tattooing for breast cancer survivors as a member of the Vinnie Myers team."

I had the implant exchange in August of 2018 and a follow-up in December of 2018. After this, I did not travel back to Mayo until August of 2019. Here is a snapshot of that visit:

Dr. Le had me disrobe from the waist up, as I had done every single time. Once she entered the room, she had me sit in her chair.

She looked at my breasts critically.

"Hmm…. there is a bit of asymmetry. I don't remember that post-surgery."

She had not seen me for a whole year, though, and I think that as a plastic surgeon, she is absolutely a perfectionist.

It was interesting because I had not really seen the asymmetry that she was talking about. To me, my breasts looked pretty good, but her comment made me question everything a bit.

"If you want, I can easily correct that for you," she said, "it would be a very easy surgery."

Doug and I looked at each other.

"You can do whatever you want, Heidi, but I think they look great."

I was a little torn, and this possibility had never entered my mind, but I am a kind of "good enough" girl in most things, and told her I was OK for now. When I need to have the implants exchanged (and I will), I will hopefully correct the asymmetry and go just a little bigger.

After a follow-up appointment at Mayo with plastic surgery, we drove the 90 miles to Mankato for an afternoon appointment at Mecca Tattoo. Doug decided to walk just a few blocks down the road for a beer while I got my nipples done. Honestly, I hardly felt anything because I have very little sensation in my foobs. It was easy to chat with Trent. The whole time I was going through reconstruction, I imagined that getting the tattoos would be this whole big deal where, at the end, I would have some huge emotional moment and feel like breast cancer was behind me. I had imagined taking the girls with me and we would all cry (or something). That feeling didn't come, though. When Trent finished his work, I was pleased with how the tattoos looked, but there was no emotional outpouring or sense that I had crossed the finish line. It was actually kind of anti-climactic. That is OK, though, a lot of life is anti-climactic, honestly. Getting my life back together turned out to be a bigger deal-more about this in the next post.

ENDING ONE JOURNEY, STARTING ANOTHER— LAST POST

Journal Entry by Heidi Edwards
September 5, 2018

It always thrills me a bit to find significance and connection in places, dates, and events. I thought about writing this post last night, but I decided to wait until today because today is September 5th. Today marks exactly fourteen months since I was diagnosed with breast cancer (July 5th, 2017). For most of that time, I was in active treatment. I want to mark this day as a day of ending. I am ending...........

- four treatments of Adriamycin and Cytoxan (two weeks apart)
- four Neulasta injections
- twelve treatments of Taxol (once every week for 12 weeks)
- a bilateral mastectomy
- drains after surgery
- 8 cycles of Xeloda (2 weeks on meds and one week off-4 pills in a.m. and 4 pills in p.m.)
- tissue expanders at the start of reconstruction
- implant surgery on 8/24/18
- velcro compression bras after each breast surgery
- a case of shingles during treatment
- hair loss (complete baldness really)
- hand and foot syndrome from the Xeloda
- lots and lots of trips to the Cancer Center
- lots and lots of trips to Mayo
- a dog bite and an updated tetanus vaccine
- I also want to mark this day as a day of starting another journey. I am starting............

- working 55% (that's what my contract states) back at the University of WI
- life as a grayhaired hot mama :)
- a life that includes daily exercise to ward off recurrence
- a Mediterranean/Paleoish diet with a low glycemic index
- daily time in devotion (not really starting, but continuing with)

I am also focusing on being DELIBERATELY GRATEFUL FOR..............

- a body that allows me to do what I want to do
- an amazing partner, Doug, who has walked beside me at one of the darkest times of my life
- precious daughters that remind me that "I am their mama and they need me."
- my sweet family (Mom, Dad, brothers, sister-in-law, and nieces and nephews who have supported us so faithfully)
- friends that have become family
- EACH BEAUTIFUL DAY with all of its hiccups and troubles and joy and laughter
- Jesus Christ, for holding me in the palm of HIS hands

Ok, I am sure that anyone still reading these posts is like, "Ok, lady, enough already." Maybe this post is overkill, but I needed to mark this day and this time and give it a formal ending. Maybe I will have to deal with cancer again. Hopefully I never will, but for now, I am closing this chapter. MOVING ON....................

"Let us (me) run with perseverance the race that is set before us (me), looking to Jesus, the pioneer and perfecter of our faith." Hebrews 12:1-2

Reflection

Moving on was easier said than done. After taking a year off from working, I was happy to be back as an adjunct English instructor at a local branch of the University of Wisconsin for Fall Term 2018. (I know how very, very lucky I was to be able to take time off.) I remember being very tired that first semester back. We had an old oversized chair and ottoman in our house that we decided to replace just a few weeks before I started back to work. Doug and the girls helped me carry both pieces of furniture from the minivan to the elevator to my NEW and UPGRADED office with a window. After each morning of teaching, I would come back and nap in the chair during my lunch break with my feet on the ottoman until I headed off to the Writing Center in the afternoon to work as a writing tutor. I was just tired. Sometimes, I felt so tired my brain even hurt. I still get like that sometimes.

That Thanksgiving, for my Mom's 70th birthday, we decided to meet in Minneapolis to celebrate Thanksgiving, and most importantly, Mom's birthday. I remember being pooped out and napping a bit each afternoon over the long weekend. My mom noticed, worried, and she called me when we were both back at home.

"I didn't want to say anything, honey, but I am worried about you. You seemed tired this weekend.. Is everything OK?"

She didn't say anything about cancer, but I knew that is what she was asking about. I get it. If one of my daughter's was recovering from cancer, I would be very alert to any real or perceived symptoms. Of course, I would be concerned about a recurrence.

"I'm fine, Mom, I usually nap a little in the afternoons," I responded. We left it at that and she did not ask me more, but I am sure she still worried. A year of treatment takes a lot out of a person, and the recovery is, for many, as long or longer than the treatment. For me at least, there was little in terms of formal support for this journey. I had one appointment with a "Nurse Navigator" who gave me a folder with some handouts and a summary of my cancer history. Post care is one area of cancer care that is lacking for many patients.

September 5, 2018 marked the end of my Caringbridge posts. I moved into "Life After Cancer". That could be a whole other book, but here are the highlights from my perspective.

LIFE AFTER CANCER—PHYSICAL CHANGES

As time has passed, I have recovered from the effects of the chemotherapy. I am much more energetic, and I don't need to nap in the afternoons. Also, my energy level is much more consistent. For the first couple of years post-treatment, I could go strong for about three days, and then I would just be wiped and need to rest on the fourth day or so. Now I am pretty much back to pre-cancer energy levels. My mom's maiden name is Petersen, and all of the Petersen's are HIGH ENERGY. I am back to "Petersen energy"-the kind of energy where you don't sit still much and "fun" is working or cleaning or just puttering around.

I have kept my hair short and gray. Initially, it was very white, but as time has passed, it has gotten darker and I am sporting a salt and pepper look. I still get asked if I want the "senior discount", but now instead of being offended, I just take it. I am my father's daughter after all and a discount is a discount.

My breasts a.k.a. foobs are fine. I am happy with them, and I don't need to wear a bra unless I want to or unless I am wearing something that is very close-fitting to even out the slight asymmetry. I do wish my foobs were slightly bigger, but the next time I need an implant exchange, I may just shoot for a slightly bigger version of what I currently have.

I still feel like my cognitive function is diminished. I love language and words, and sometimes, even now, I struggle to find the right words and/or I am not satisfied with how I articulate something. I feel like I am (and I ACTUALLY am) more forgetful—especially when recalling names or places. Chemo brain is a real thing, but thankfully, my memory has definitely improved over the past couple of years. Initially, I lost literally everything—keys, my phone, money—you name it, I lost it. Poor Doug said he was scared to put me in charge of anything. That has gotten much better, but as stated in the first sentence of this paragraph, it is still noticeable and still something I mourn.

I have some neuropathy in my hands and feet, especially when they get cold. I doubt it will get better, and I just hope it doesn't get worse.

LIFE AFTER CANCER—FAMILY UPDATE

The girls don't like to talk about cancer, and I don't talk about it with them very often. Grace recently graduated from high school (May 2021) and at her graduation party, we put together a table that represented her and displayed pieces of her life that were important to her. This is a pretty common practice here in the Midwest, and maybe all over the United States? On her table, nestled next to artwork, photos, two of her favorite pairs of shoes, and many other items there were a few nods to breast cancer-a pink scarf from a Susan G. Komen run and a Stand up to Cancer bracelet she wore when I was going through treatment. It was a quiet acknowledgement of cancer's impact on her life.

Avery and Lauren have a tender place for what cancer means to families. Last year, one of their classmates' mom was going through cancer and they tried their best to support her via meals, gifts, a t-shirt purchase, and just a general awareness and empathy. Another classmate lost her mom to cancer and they cried. They don't say much anymore about our family's journey with cancer though.

Doug and I don't talk about cancer much anymore either. During the year that I was going through treatment and for quite a while after, cancer was the focus of most of our conversations. Now, we have moved on to other things—the girls, our jobs, the cabin, the pandemic. In the summer of 2019, both Doug and Grace had very difficult summers that extended into trying autumns. I feel like they both experienced a bit of PTSD, but we got through that season. I wonder if this is common in other families. When caregivers/family members finally have permission to fall apart, maybe they do? I haven't explored this theory with too many people, but I am curious.

LIFE AFTER CANCER-MY WORK LIFE

Immediately post-cancer, I worked for one academic year at our local branch of the University of Wisconsin, a role I had been in for ten years. I was ready for a change, though, and when a job opened up working with K-5 second language learners, I decided to give it a whirl and leave post-secondary learners for a while. Right now, I am in my third year as an English Language Interventionist at an elementary school in north central Wisconsin. It has been a great switch, and one of the best parts is being able to work with families. Working in this role has been very fulfilling for me, especially during the pandemic.

LIFE AFTER CANCER- MY EMOTIONAL STATE

I don't worry about a recurrence daily as I did initially post-treatment. I still see Dr. Anand every six months, and I believe I will do that until I am five years from diagnosis. Each time that I go in for a check-up, I feel a little sick to my stomach. The other sucky thing about this kind of cancer (TNBC) is that there really is no "test" to assure that a patient is cancer-free. When I go in for a check-up, there are no scans or tests or bloodwork. The nurse asks me a series of questions and Dr. Anand does a physical exam. A recurrence would mostly likely be caught based on the existence of a symptom. I realize that by the time a symptom showed up, it would be a very worrisome prognostic sign. For example, if I began having double vision or severe headaches or dizziness, the concern would be a metastasis to the brain. Even in a scenario like that, though, there is still hope. There is always hope.

Bottom line......

There are no guarantees, but that is true for most (all) of life. At a certain point, you just have to let go and live in faith and not fear. There is no other option. And what if the cancer does come back? Again, the only option would be living in faith and not fear. And what if death was imminent? Again-the only answer would be faith and not fear. This is easier said than done, I know, but as a believer and Christ-follower, I put my faith and trust in Jesus.

Sometimes, I get angry with myself because some of the changes I made during cancer and realizations I had have faded with time. For example, I can easily get frustrated with the girls and Doug, and I am not as patient as I was three years ago when I had just finished treatment. I can get annoyed by little things like a broken garage door or waiting on hold with the internet company. I have also gotten more lax with my diet.

All of these things make me frustrated with myself, and I worry that I am wasting the lessons of cancer. I try to remind myself what cancer taught me and to keep those lessons more forefront. Maybe that is the challenge post-cancer—moving forward, but at the same time being changed by the experience and not wasting (not sure that is the right word) the experience.

How Has The Experience of Cancer Changed Me?

I wrote this narrative as a way to document my experiences and to connect with others who have had, are having, or will have a similar experience. Writing is a way of creating meaning and documenting our humanity. As I have mentioned a number of times, my experience is not unique; my purpose in writing is not to draw attention to myself or elevate myself as some amazing person who survived breast cancer. I am not amazing; I just had breast cancer. I am writing to sort through and express the complicated and emotional experience that breast cancer was for me. As I sift through all of it, these are the lessons that I hold firmly in my hands.

Perspective

The biggest thing that breast cancer has given me is perspective.

When I am tempted to wallow in self-pity (still do quite a bit because I am human) or get angry or frustrated about something inconsequential (still do quite a bit because I am human), I remind myself of the weight that cancer was. I remind myself of how it felt at the beginning, when I didn't know if I would respond to treatment or if I would go home to be with Jesus. I remind myself that this current trial is small and manageable; I remind myself that it could be so much worse. I remind myself that today's worry, while still real and still right there, is something I can deal with.

I want to speak to and acknowledge the fact that some people themselves or those they love do not survive health crises, and I am sure that their perspective has been mightily changed by the journey they have walked. I cannot speak to that perspective right now, but in reading about other people's stories, most of those on that journey speak of a deeper gratitude and appreciation for each day and for the love and kindness of family and friends. Most speak of more intentional living.

I also want to speak to the fact that many people have health struggles that they live with forever or love and care for people with health struggles much more serious than the one I faced. I am not in a position to speak about how those individuals navigate life.

Never Enough Time

I remember when I was first diagnosed, I thought.......I hope that I just get to do _____ or see _____. In 2019, Mom, Dad, our family, and my niece, Katelyn all went on a river boat cruise down the Rhine River. I started planning the trip a full year before, in 2018. I had not even finished the Xeloda (oral chemo) yet, and the trip was to be, for me, a celebration of surviving cancer. I even got my sweet Papa Lou to go! He couldn't say no to his daughter's request after a year of dealing with the shit storm that was breast cancer. It was something to look forward to and dream about. The whole year before we actually made that trip, I prayed and hoped that I would be able to go.

After that, I prayed that I would be around for Grace's graduation. (Of course, I have hoped and prayed for a whole host of other little things.) Grace graduated and I feel much more optimistic about my future, but still, I realize that for most people, there is always a desire for more time. Even though you reach one milestone, it isn't enough. You always ache and yearn for more time. THERE IS NEVER ENOUGH TIME.

I Feel Your Pain

Another change in me is a deepened empathy for the suffering of others. Cancer has given me empathy, not only for those dealing with cancer, but for suffering and pain in general. The older I get and the more suffering and pain I see in the lives of others, the more I realize that there is rarely anything I can do to "fix" or "change" the hardship. It seems to me that the only thing I can do is care and walk beside the person or people who are struggling. This is another lesson I need to work very diligently on to make sure it stays in the forefront.

People Are So Good/We Are All So Intimately Connected

People are really so good. I have never felt as loved in my life as I did when I was going through treatment. I felt pure love, complete love from so many people. One example of love that completely stood out to me came from the woman who was grooming Louise at the time. I know that she had very, very little, but at Christmas time, when I went in to pick up Louise (our dog) after her grooming, the woman handed me a $20 bill. At this point, I had been in treatment since July and she knew about the cancer. She said, "I want to give you this. You can use it to help pay for Louise's grooming or maybe buy yourself something." I tried to refuse, but she was insistent, and so I accepted the money and that gift in particular made me teary. Another woman, the mother of one of my friends, sent me three crisp $20 bills in the mail. The lunch lady where my kids went to elementary school sent me a $25.00 gift card to a local restaurant called 2510. The list goes on and on. I read a quote that I think I referenced earlier, but it is so applicable here and it definitely bears repeating. "Healing is receiving love." I received so much love, and I did heal, so I am pretty sure there is something to that. Most humans hate to see the suffering of others, and they do what they can to alleviate/address/acknowledge that suffering.

Life is So Beautiful

There are times, usually when I am with my girls or Doug, when the richness and sanctity of life just wells up inside me to such a degree that I can literally feel it. This awareness of life's beauty and richness is something that is so easy to take for granted until you understand that life and living do not go on forever. When you realize they are finite, that awareness is almost heart-breaking. For most of us (myself included), mindfulness is rarely practiced. When I was thinking about this, I thought about Emily in Thorton Wilder's play, "Our Town" and her powerful words. Wilder expresses all these ideas in such a powerful way.

(Right after I wrote this section of my narrative, Lauren and Avery had an "Our Town" unit for their 10th grade English language arts class. I don't think that is just coincidental.)

In case you have never read the play or if it has been a looong time, here is a quick summary. In Act One, we meet the two main characters of the play, Emily Webb and George Gibbs and their families who live in Grover's Corner, NH in the year 1901. The act ends with the discovery that Emily and George like each other. In Act Two, despite last minute nerves and some "letting go of dreams" to be together, George and Emily get married. In Act Three, we learn (from the Stage Manager who serves as the narrator), that Emily has died in childbirth. The deceased Emily realizes she is able to relive certain days of her life. The other deceased townspeople warn her not to go back to the past, but she ignores their warnings, and decides to relive her twelfth birthday. The experience leaves her heartbroken because she realizes that most people live life without appreciating it. Her lines below express this so eloquently that the play is still taught in high schools and performed almost 100 years later.

EMILY: "Oh, earth, you're too wonderful for anybody to realize you."

EMILY: "Does anyone ever realize life while they live it...every, every minute?"

STAGE MANAGER: "No. Saints and poets maybe...they do some."

EMILY: "Let's really look at one another!...It goes so fast. We don't have time to look at one another. I didn't realize. So all that was going on and we never noticed... Wait! One more look. Good-bye, Good-bye world. Good-bye, Grover's Corners....Mama and Papa. Good-bye to clocks ticking....and Mama's sunflowers. And food and coffee. And new ironed dresses and hot baths....and sleeping and waking up. Oh, earth, you are too wonderful for anybody to realize you. Do any human beings ever realize life while they live it—every, every minute?"

If I had to narrow down what cancer has taught me to one single lesson, it would absolutely be this—to be present and grateful for the ordinary. From the right vantage point, the ordinary becomes extraordinary.

A NOTE ON THE PROVIDERS WHO LITERALLY SAVED MY LIFE

Two things strike me as I edit my words and reflect on my caregivers. First of all, most of the physicians who cared for me, not just my oncologist, were not born in the United States. In fact, some of them went to medical school in other countries and then came to the United States to complete their residencies and eventually practice. Their presence in this country has changed the course of LITERALLY THOUSANDS OF LIVES. Where would the patients they have served be if they had not immigrated here? This fact is especially meaningful to me as I have dedicated a great deal of my life to teaching English to speakers of other languages.

Secondly, interestingly enough, three of my physicians in Wausau and almost all of them at Mayo were women. According to Wikipedia, women were 9% of total medical school enrollment in 1969; presently women make up slightly more than half of those in medical school. That, my friends, is powerful. I was equally well cared for by my male and female physicians. I was equally impressed by my male and female physicians. I appreciated the perspective of both my male and female physicians. I am glad I had breast cancer in 2017 and not fifty years earlier, in 1967, because I had the opportunity to glean wisdom from and to receive care from **both** men and women.

To all my health care providers, thank you for saving my life.

WORKS CITED

"American Cancer Society." *"Tips for Healthy Eating After Cancer Treatment*, American Cancer Society, 9 June 2020, cancer.org. Accessed 26 September 2021.

American Cancer Society. ""Breast MRI."" *"Breast MRI"*, American Cancer Society. 3 October 2019, cancer.org/cancer/breast-cancer/ screening-tests-and-early-detection/breast-mri-scans.html. Accessed 14 September 2021.

American Cancer Society. ""Eating Well During Treatment."" *"Eating Well During Treatment"*, American Cancer Society, 9 June 2020, cancer. org. Accessed 26 September 2021.

American Cancer Society. ""Triple Negative Breast Cancer."" *"Triple Negative Breast Cancer"*, American Cancer Society, 27 January 2021, https:www.cancer.org/cancer/breast-cancer/about/types-of-breast-cancer/triple-negative.html. Accessed 13 September 2021.

American Psychological Association. "Flashbulb Memory." *dictionary. apa.org*, APA, 2020 Unknown 2020, https://dictionary.apa.org/flash-bulb-memory. Accessed 12 September 2021.

Bowler, Kate. *Everything Happens For A Reason and Other LIes I've Loved*. London, Random House Trade Paperbacks., 2019.

CancerCare Co-Payment Assistance Foundation, 2021, cancercare.org/ copayfoundation.

Canterbury Health Laboratories. ""Cell Block-Cytology."" *"Cell Block-Cytology"*, Canterbury Health Laboratories, Unknown Unknown 2013, http://labnet.health.nz/testmanager/index.php?fuseaction=-main.DisplayTest&testid=14. Accessed 12 September 2021.

Christians in Action. *CIA Cookbook*. Eldora, Iowa, St. Paul Lutheran Church, 1990.

Christofferson, MS, Travis. *Tripping Over the Truth*. White River Junction, VT, Chelsea Green Publishing, 2017.

Girard, Vickie. *There's No Place Like Hope: A Guide to Beating Cancer in Mind-Sized Bites*. Seattle, Compendium Publishing and Communications, 2008.

Health Clinics USA Corporation. "Changing the Face of Cancer Treatment-Care Oncology." *www.careoncology.com*, Care Oncology. Accessed 28 September 2021.

Ingram, Deputy Managing Editor, Ian. "Residual Breast Cancer Tool Highly Prognostic After Neoadjuvant Tx-Tumor burden calculator predicted long-term outcomes in all breast cancer subtypes." MedPage Today, 14 December 2019, http://www.medpagetoday.com/meetingcoverage/sabcs/83906.

Kalamian, Miriam. *Keto for Cancer*. White River Junction, Vermont, Chelsea Green Publishing, 2017.

Klett, Leach Marie Ann. ""Stroke Survivor Katherine Wolf on Finding God In Suffering: 'There's Hidden Treasure In Darkness.'"" *Christian Post*, May 17, 2020. *christian post.com*. Accessed 17 September 2021.

Leukemia and Lymphoma Society. "Leukemia and Lymphoma Society." *www.lls.org*, 2021.

Lewis, C.S. *"Mere Christianity"*. vol. pages 175-176, New York, Touchstone, 1996.

Mecca Tattoo, LLC. 2021, www.meccatattoo.com.

Miranda, Lin-manuel. ""Who Lives? Who Dies? Who Tells Your Story."" *Hamilton*, Lin-manuel Miranda, 2015.

National Cancer Institute. "NCI Dictionaries-Dictionary of Cancer Terms." *NCI Dictionaries-Dictionary of Cancer Terms*, National Cancer Institute, Unknown Unknown Unknown, cancer.gov/publications/dictionaries/cancer-terms/def/port. Accessed 15 September 2021.

Nordeman, Nichole, and Jen Hatmaker. ""Find Your Elephant Tribe."" *the well*, The Well Team, Unknown Unknown Unknown, faithforgirlsbygirls.com/the-elephant-story-by-jen-hatmaker. Accessed 16 September 2021.

PAN Foundation. "PAN Foundation." *www.panfoundation.org*, 2021.

Paris, Twila. ""How Beautiful The Hands that Served."" *Cry for the Desert*, 1990.

Prijatel, Patricia. *Surviving Triple Negative Breast Cancer: Hope, Treatment, and Recovery*. USA, Oxford University Press, Inc., 2014.

Shakespeare, William. *Hamlet*. Edited by George Richard Hibbard, Oxford University Press, 2008. *Google Books*.

Stefanie de Groot, Rieneke T. Lugtenberg, Danielle Cohen, Marij J. P. Welters, Ilina Ehsan, Maaike P. G. Vreeswijk, Vincent T. H. B. M. Smit, Hiltje de Graaf, Joan B. Heijns, Johanneke E. A. Portielje, Agnes J. van de Wouw, Alex L. T. Imholz, Lonneke W. Ke. "Fasting mimicking diet as an adjunct to neoadjuvant chemotherapy for breast cancer in the multicentre randomized phase 2 DIRECT trial." Nature Communications, 23 June 2020, https://www.nature.com/articles/s41467-020-16138-3#citeas. Accessed 27 September 2021.

Taste of Home. "Favorite Chicken Pot Pie." Taste of Home, Unknown Unknown Unknown. Accessed 28 September 2021.

Wagner, Holly. *Find Your Brave: Courage to Stand Strong When the Waves Crash In*. New York City, Crown Publishing Group, 2016.

Wilder, Thornton. *"Our Town: A Play in Three Acts"*. 1938.